The Desperate Woman's Guide to Fitness will:

- Get you off of your butt and into a fitness program.
- Make **any** fitness program work.
- Make your dust-covered collection of fitness, nutrition, and exercise books start working for you.
- Improve your sex life (and, of course, your jewelry).
- Show you the sensible way to stay fit for life.
- Assure you that complaining about working out is normal and actually good for your health.

The Desperate Woman's Guide to Fitness won't:

- Offer a six-week miracle program. (**Any** positve changes in eating and exercise habits will lead to improvement in six weeks. The miracle is to make the changes permanent!)
- Tell you how to lose forty pounds in four days.
- Solve your daughter-in-law problems.
- Cause mood swings or memory loss.

The Desperate Woman's Guide to Fitness

by

Ellen Morrow

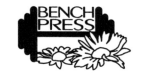

BENCH PRESS

Los Angeles, California

The Desperate Woman's Guide to Fitness
by Ellen Morrow

Published by: Bench Press 1997
P.O. Box 571715
Tarzana, California 91357

Illustrations by: Carole Raschella
Book design and typography by: Randi Rose
Cover design by: Paul Chepikian
Cover photo by: Jerry Fredrick

Library of Congress Catalog Card No. 97-093484

Publisher's Cataloguing-in-Publication
(Provided by Quality Books, Inc.)

Morrow, Ellen Potter.
    The desperate woman's guide to fitness : by Ellen Morrow — 1st ed.
    p. cm.
    ISBN: 0-9656964-4-8

    1. Physical Fitness for women. 2. Aging — Humor. I. Title
GV482.M67 1997   613.7'045
                                      QBI97-40475

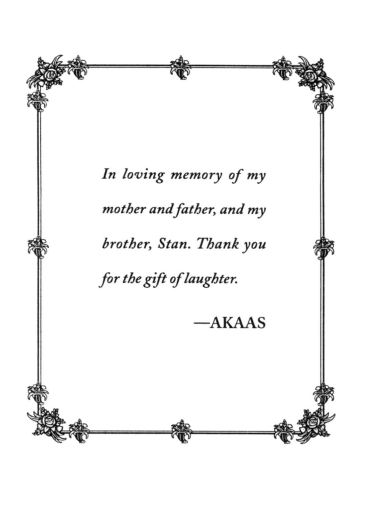

In loving memory of my mother and father, and my brother, Stan. Thank you for the gift of laughter.

—AKAAS

ACKNOWLEDGMENTS

A very loving thank you to my husband, Doug, and to my daughters, Jennifer, Nicole, and Danielle, for their love and understanding and for being a constant source of material.

My gratitude to Alice Noble and Mish Kaplan for their hours of patient editing and for always being available when I needed a rational head, and to Audrey Rubin for fact checking.

Thank you to Carole Raschella, Randi Rose, and Paul Chepikian for creating such a wonderful setting for my words.

Sincere appreciation to all of my desperate friends and relatives for their encouragement and support and for listening to me complain.

TABLE OF CONTENTS

	Preface	11
Chapter 1	Who Is This Desperate Woman?	13
Chapter 2	The Truth About Desperation	17
Chapter 3	The Truth About Aging–the Over Forty Gang	23
Chapter 4	The Truth About Fitness	27
Chapter 5	Stop the Treadmill–I Want to Get Off	31
Chapter 6	Aerobic Alternatives–Pick Your Poison	39
	Jogging	40
	Stairclimbing	42
	Walking	43
	Aerobics Classes	45
	Stationary Equipment	49
	Triathlons	51
	Martial Arts	52
	Hiking	54
	Biking	60
Chapter 7	Real Women Don't Iron–They Pump It	65
Chapter 8	Flexibility Over Forty–Fact or Fiction?	83
Chapter 9	You Are What You Eat–Except When You Have PMS	93
Chapter 10	Taming the Stress Monster	109
Chapter 11	Help! Where Do I Begin?	117
Chapter 12	Your Home Away From Home	123
Chapter 13	Mistakes	131
Chapter 14	Motivation	141
Chapter 15	Is That All There Is? Five Extra Keys to Fitness	153
Chapter 16	In Conclusion	167
	Glossary	171

PREFACE

As an over forty (way over forty) bodybuilder, I have been approached by countless women over the years seeking advice about health and fitness. This book is my answer to their questions about shaping up, staying motivated, and confronting the many challenges of aging.

The older I've gotten and the more women I've spoken to in the gym, the more I've come to realize that we're all fighting the same battles. I've also learned that our most effective weapon against desperation, aside from commiserating with each other, is the ability to laugh at the things that we simply cannot fix. It's desperation tempered with a healthy dose of humor.

About the Text

Within the general text I've indicated specific **hints** that will make the job easier, **good news** that will cheer you up, as well as **warnings** that will insure safety. I've also included several **personal anecdotes**. They're italicized so they can easily be skipped, but reading about my experiences, many of them disastrous, may be just what it takes to get you over the rough spots, to help you cope with feelings of discouragement or intimidation.

Chapter 1

Who Is This Desperate Woman?

In the early eighties, muscular women, particularly muscular mothers of three, were not exactly in vogue. Doing aerobics was okay, jogging was acceptable, but pumping iron put you into some sort of lunatic fringe group. For a natural born klutz like myself, it was an even stranger exercise choice. I used to tell people that I was going to the mall because I was too embarrassed to admit that I was lifting weights. As my muscles grew, I blamed the development on heavy shopping bags. Obviously, with this attitude, entering the world of women's bodybuilding was not something that I'd ever planned on doing. Like so much in life, it was a result of circumstances beyond my control.

Raised as a devout non-athlete in Syracuse, New York, I had so many excuses for getting out of gym class that even the teachers were impressed. Uncoordinated and disinclined toward any form of physical activity, my idea of exercise was watching *Bowling for Dollars* with my family. To be fair, my parents did send me for ballet lessons, but I think it was only their desperate attempt to buy me some poise and grace. They claimed to be very proud of my progress, so I could never understand why they showed up at my recitals using assumed names and wearing fake noses with mustaches attached.

Throughout high school and college I enrolled in the minimum number and the easiest physical education classes that I could possibly find. For instance, I took a class in college called rhythmic gymnastics, not to be confused with real gymnastics or the Olympic event of the same name. We'd run around the gym on tiptoe, waving scarves or twirling little rings. It was like a remedial class for the athletically challenged.

It was only when I became pregnant with my first child that I realized it might be time for some genuine exercise. I began swimming laps, a logical choice since my husband and I had recently moved to California, and since I was starting to bear a distinct resemblance to Moby Dick. By my ninth month I was so huge that people were trying to harpoon me in the pool, but thanks to the swimming, my body rebounded in record time.

During my second pregnancy I turned to tennis (at which I was truly terrible) and bike riding. For the third, I signed up for ballet and psychological counseling since my older girls were only two and five. It was also during my third pregnancy that a life changing event took place.

Seven months pregnant, I was a passenger in a head-on automobile accident. My head hit the dashboard with enough force to fracture my skull and shatter virtually every bone in my face. Even more critically, a tangerine-size blood clot formed on my brain. Within days, I underwent a nine hour operation which included the initial phase of plastic surgery and a craniotomy to remove the clot. Two weeks later, my daughter Danielle was born, a full month early but miraculously healthy and hardy.

Over the next few years, I was in and out of the hospital as the long, grueling process of facial reconstruction was completed. Due to the surgeries, associated periods of recuperation, and emotional strain, I ended up as a ninety pound weakling with a bad attitude.

Around the time that I was feeling severely depressed about my physical condition, my husband and I attended a charity event at a health club. Intrigued by the weight training machines, I bought a membership to the club and began a personal effort at rehabilitation.

After a few months, bored and disenchanted with the machines, I switched to free weights, receiving guidance from someone who quite proudly informed me that he was a bodybuilder. A little confused, since the only bodybuilder I was familiar with was a hair care product, I nonetheless accepted his advice because he was the strongest person I'd ever met. With his encouragement, I embarked upon a more in-depth exercise regimen and eventually gathered up the courage to trade the safety of the plush health club for the more serious atmosphere of a hard-core weight lifting gym.

After recovering from the initial culture shock and overcoming my fear of the huge, muscle-bound members, I worked out harder than ever and eventually grew to love that place. Several months later (I'm still not sure how it happened), I found myself in training for a bodybuilding competition.

As a quiet, traditional carpool mom still carrying the physical and emotional scars of the accident, competing in that first show was probably the most difficult thing I'd ever attempted—not to mention, the weirdest. The physical preparation was intense and gratifying, but pumping up backstage and then stepping onto the posing platform was an almost overwhelming challenge. I just kept telling myself that if I could do it, I could do anything. The competition became a symbol of my recovery—something that I had to accomplish in order to regain my self-esteem and prove to myself that I was really okay.

I was in for a big surprise when I collected my trophy (aside from the surprise that I'd even won a trophy). I wanted to compete again. I'm not sure if it was the sense of achievement, the excitement, or the applause (probably the applause, something that I'd never received for cleaning the toilet or cooking dinner), but I was hooked.

Despite my husband's initial reservations and a severe case of stage fright, I began entering other shows and, allow me to brag, winning titles such as Ms. Venice Beach, Ms. Southern California, and Ms. Western States. When anabolic steroids infiltrated the sport, I bowed out but continued training. In 1989 I discovered a relatively new organization that not only held all natural (drug-free) shows but that also had a masters category for women over forty. This was right up my alley—middle-aged women who weren't on drugs! I jumped at the chance to get back into competition and won several new titles including the masters divisions of the Natural California, the Natural National, and the Natural Universe.

Still pumping iron after all these years, I currently reside in Southern California with my husband and either one, two, or three of our grown daughters who take turns moving in and out of the house.

Chapter 2

The Truth
About Desperation

MOST SANE WOMEN HATE TO EXERCISE, BUT SANITY IS NO EXCUSE

For years, I've been conducting an informal study on the attitudes of women, particularly women over the age of forty, as they work out. Through astute observation and even more astute eavesdropping, I've found that most of them hate it. Whether they're casual exercisers dropping in to catch up on the latest gossip, or serious athletes in training for competition, they bitch about everything imaginable. If I didn't know better, I'd assume they were being blackmailed into working out. Come to think of it, it is a form of blackmail, only cellulite can't talk.

Many people assume that because I've been a competitive bodybuilder since the dawn of time, that I live to work out. Let me clear up this misconception immediately. I'd rather be curling my eyelashes than curling a dumbbell, and I prefer bench sitting at the beach to bench pressing in the gym. Like everyone else, I exercise because I have to, and I complain constantly while I'm doing it.

Looking for a more in-depth analysis of all this negativity, I turned to my in-house experts (my daughters) to ask them why they thought women hated to exercise. In unison, they chorused, "Are you kidding? Working out sucks." Intrigued by their insight, I pressed further, "What exactly sucks about it?" Without missing a beat, they replied, "It hurts. You sweat and smell bad while you're doing it. Leotards are uncomfortable and make you look fat. And you never feel like you're making any progress so you get depressed." Mind you, this analysis comes from three young women who exercise regularly, look attractive with wet hair, and can try on bathing suits without getting suicidal.

THE TRUTH DOESN'T ALWAYS HURT

Many women on the threshold of a fitness program are in trouble before they even buy a gym bag because they don't really know what to expect. Pumped up by media hype and delusional friends, they labor under the misconception that they're going to love getting into shape. They listen to glowing reports about the joys of a fitness lifestyle and expect that after a few tofu patties and a jog around the block, they're going to experience some sort of religious conversion. Disillusioned when all they experience is fatigue, boredom, and a few sore muscles, they toss their leotards in the rag bag and try to get refunds on health club fees.

Women would stand a much better chance for success if they were told the truth—there's a big difference between the process and the results. Doing it doesn't insure that you're going to love it, but once you get going it's very difficult to stop, and the end product is usually worth the effort—sort of like childbirth.

Sure, the idea of improving your health and appearance while enjoying a longer and more productive life is enough to make you giddy, but if you think that being compelled to do regular exercise and monitor your eating is a barrel of laughs, you'd probably love prison. It may be satisfying to know that you can stay on a treadmill for fifteen minutes without hallucinating and challenging to see if you can go for a week without chocolate, but it's certainly not fun. That's why people are always looking for ways around it. If I had a dollar for every time I've heard someone say, "There's got to be an easier way," I could afford so much plastic surgery that I wouldn't have to exercise. Trust me, if there was an easier way, I'd be doing it.

You don't have to throw in the towel if you're not thrilled with aerobics and sweat and greaseless french fries. You're not some sort of dismal failure who's doomed to a life of unhealthy excess. You're normal. You can take heart in the knowledge that if you're realistic, persistent, and able to ignore annoying fitness fanatics, you may eventually learn to like what you're doing, or maybe not hate it quite so much. At the very least, you'll have developed some good habits that are just as difficult to break as the bad ones.

THE QUESTION: WHY DO WOMEN EXERCISE?

You may be asking yourself, "If so many women hate to exercise, why are millions of them doing it?" Good question, and for the longest time I racked my brain trying to figure out the answer. There had to be a reason that women of all sizes and shapes were grunting through weight lifting sessions, fighting over treadmills, and exerting themselves like construction workers, doing things they'd normally pay people to do for them. Somewhere in all of the madness, there had to be a logical explanation.

19

I considered the standard motivations:

- weight problems
- health considerations
- lack of interesting hobbies
- excuse to get out of the house
- divorce
- hormone imbalance
- brainwashing

However, none of them seemed adequate to explain the tremendous expense of time and energy and the stoic consumption of really boring food.

THE ANSWER: THEY DO IT BECAUSE THEY'RE DESPERATE

The answer finally came to me, as many great revelations do, while I was drying my hair. (I think it has something to do with the effect of the heat on my brain.) Like Einstein, who coincidentally also had a rather full head of hair, I discovered the answer to one of the great mysteries of the universe; we stuff ourselves into strange outfits and engage in an even stranger array of physical activities because we're desperate! Desperate to keep from feeling old and out of shape. Desperate to hold on to our figures, to keep our cellulite under control, and to prove that we still have what it takes, if we could only remember what that was. In short, we're so desperate that we'll try almost anything if we think it might work (and you wonder why the ThighMaster is such a popular item).

I can hear it now. Some of you are asking, "Who does this know-it-all think she is calling me desperate?" You claim that you're self-assured, have no interest whatsoever in exercising and eating right, and that no amount of begging or threatening is going to change your mind. When you see an aerobics queen prancing around the market in her leotard and tights, you want to run her over with your cart. When you see one sporting a sweat band as if it's a merit badge, you want to snap it on her forehead like a rubber band.

Let me break it to you gently. You can protest all you like, but sooner or later you're going to be involved in some sort of workout program. Curiosity, guilt, self-loathing, vanity, tipping the scales at two hundred pounds—something is going to get you to the gym, and desperation is going to make you stay.

It's inevitable. Show me an exercise arena with "mature" (euphemism alert) women working out, and I'll show you desperation. It's universal, it's highly contagious, and it's tenacious. Once it gets hold of you, it never lets go.

This isn't necessarily a bad thing because desperation can be an endless source of motivation. It can get you out of a rut and into a gym. It can get you to stop whining about the way you look and feel and to take some positive action instead. Desperation also gives you an instant bond with millions of other women who feel exactly the same way you do. Together you can find the means to combat the symptoms which made you feel this way in the first place.

QUIZ: ARE YOU A DESPERATE WOMAN?

Still feeling very insulted and defensive at being called desperate (which probably means that you are)? Still in total denial? The following quiz should clarify matters for you. Simply answer **true** or **false** to each statement to find out where you stand.

1. I'm over forty.
2. I use the TV remote control because I get tired if I have to keep getting up to change the channel.
3. I have no life.
4. I have difficulty walking because my thighs chafe.
5. I wear slip-on shoes because I can't get close enough to my feet to tie laces.
6. I've been on and off so many exercise and diet programs that I've lost count.
7. I avoid the butter/margarine controversy by cooking with lard.
8. I wear spandex in public.
9. People say I look very mature for my age.
10. When I went for a physical, my doctor couldn't stop laughing.
11. I'd pass up a close encounter with Mel Gibson in order to attend

a lecture on menopause, osteoporosis, or bladder prolapse.
12. The last time I reached my ideal weight was in eighth grade.
13. I wouldn't know a good night's sleep if I had one.
14. I live in a climate where mukluks and an over-size parka are not always appropriate attire.
15. I'd cover my body with bacon fat and wrap it in cellophane if I thought it would get rid of cellulite.
16. Even though I'm thin, my arms and legs flap when I walk.
17. I insist that they evacuate the store when I try on bathing suits.
18. I turn out the lights and cover the mirrors when I have sex, even if I'm alone.
19. I weigh myself several times a day, hoping to get a number that I like.
20. After I pull back the skin on my face to see how I'd look with a facelift, I lift up my breasts to see if I can remember where they used to go.
21. I believe that ice cream is the number one cure for depression.
22. I'm reading this book and taking this dumb quiz.

We don't even have to discuss your answers because they're personal and probably none of my business. Suffice it to say that if you responded true to two or more—welcome to the wonderful world of desperation where almost anything is possible because you have nothing to lose.

Chapter 3

The Truth About Aging:
The Over Forty Gang

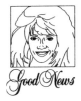

In case you read the words "over forty," got completely turned off, and don't even want to deal with this section, let me give you the good news right up front. Changing your lifestyle can have very positive effects on the aging process. It can:
- *prevent an increase in blood pressure*
- *prevent or slow down the development of osteoporosis*
- *prevent an increase in body fat and body weight*
- *help you retain normal brain function*
- *help you retain muscle tone and strength*
- *help you retain flexibility*

Now that I have your attention, brace yourself and read on.

THE TURNING POINT

Although the need for exercise and the basic tenets of fitness apply to women of all ages, I'm addressing myself primarily to women over forty because forty is a major turning point in terms of desperation. Believe it or not, there are some women in their teens, twenties, and even thirties who think it's fun to work out. Exercise is less effort for them and recuperation is faster. They can do it if they're in the mood or skip it if they're not, without doing too much harm. Being sedentary will effect them in the long run, but they can probably get away with it for quite awhile. Simply getting out of bed in the morning and breathing may be enough to keep them in shape. As a bonus, with a little extra exertion, they stand a better than even chance of attaining the body that they'd like.

When you're over forty, weight control is more difficult and exercise is harder. Recuperation is slower, plus you're more prone to injuries and probably won't heal as fast as you used to. To add insult to injury, the only way that you're going to get the twenty year old body of your dreams is to kidnap him or buy him a drink.

But if you don't exercise, your body is going to fall apart right before your eyes. Actually it isn't right before your eyes. I've watched mine to see if I could pinpoint the exact moment when parts were starting to sag. It seemed to me that if I could catch them in the act, I might be able to do some major damage control. Sorry to report, so far my attempts have been futile.

The last time I went for a check-up, I was sitting in a waiting room where I couldn't help but notice a conspicuous display of pamphlets labeled "Life After 45." As if that wasn't bad enough, the covers featured photos of women who were wearing polyester blouses, bermuda shorts, and pearls. To top it off, they all looked so constipated, they would have been shoo-ins for laxative ads.

Not wanting to broadcast my age, I surreptitiously glanced at some of the topics: estrogen therapy, menopause, hysterectomy... and then fainted. When I came to, I gasped to a woman across the room, "Have you seen these things?" With tears in her eyes, she replied, "Why do you think I'm sitting all the way over here?" When I confronted the doctor, he said that he'd never noticed how prominently displayed they were and promised to move them. For someone who'd never had a hot flash, he was quite sensitive.

There are other reasons that I see the forties as a turning point. At forty people began saying to me, "You're in such fabulous shape," but before I could blush and say thank you, would add, "for a woman your age." Around the same period, someone at the gym, who was young enough to have acne for the first time, confided that I was his older woman fantasy. Even though I wasn't really sure how to take that, I was a little disappointed when he didn't invite me to his prom.

NO EXCUSES, PLEASE

No matter how you look at it, it's more difficult to stay in shape as you get older. Yet, in many ways it's more important because your health is at stake as well as your vanity. Of course, if you enjoy watching your breasts hit your waist and your rear end scrape the back of your knees, you don't have to bother. If you get a kick out of passing out when you walk up a flight of stairs or run for a bus, you don't have to waste your time. If broken bones and sore joints don't phase you, you can sit back and relax. Your body will do the rest.

IT'S NEVER TOO LATE

Don't tell me it's too late for you to start. We all should have started exercising at birth if we wanted to stay ahead of the game, but who has that much foresight? No matter how old you are, regular exercise is an important factor in "staying younger," both physically and psychologically.

I've spoken to women in their sixties and seventies who have increased their energy and strength by getting into modified workout programs. Daily walks and light weight training have given them a new lease on life. As an added benefit, at that age they actually enjoy exercising because they're so thankful they can still do it!

If women can make progress at that stage of life, imagine what you can do by starting in your forties or even fifties. You'll be light years ahead of the game. You'll be so toned that the twenty year old body of your dreams may come running after you. Unfortunately, he'll only want to know how you manage to look so terrific at your age so that he can pass the secret on to his girlfriend.

Chapter 4

The Truth About Fitness

WHAT DOES IT MEAN TO BE FIT?

Now that you've bravely come out of the closet and admitted that you're over forty and desperate, you have to do something about it. Assuming that your general goal is to get fit, the first step is to determine exactly what being fit means to you. If you don't want to waste your time on this type of discussion and just want to get to the nuts and bolts of an actual fitness regimen, skip this section. Better yet, jog in place and eat rice cakes while you read it.

The dictionary defines "fit" as "having the necessary qualities." Ask yourself what qualities you consider to be necessary. Which of the following concerns you more?

A. Depressing medical data like how soon your heart is going to give out and how much cholesterol you have in your body or
B. Making sure that your butt doesn't hit the ground before you do

Which are you more preoccupied with?

A. When you're going to die or
B. Making sure that you look your best when it's time to go

Hint

If you'd cancel an emergency appendectomy before you'd cancel a hair appointment, your answer to each question is "B". By the way, the dictionary also defines "fit" as "healthy and strong," but that's number three on the list. Don't be put off if your goals are a little more shallow. There's a lot to be said for vanity, especially if it causes you to improve your lifestyle.

WHAT ARE THE BASICS OF GETTING FIT?

Despite all of the often confusing and conflicting information about exercise and nutrition, getting fit is not that complicated. It involves certain basic components that should be incorporated into your lifestyle if you want to give the twenty and thirty somethings a run for their money. These components may be handled in different ways, but together they make up the framework for a solid fitness program.

- Aerobic exercise to improve cardiovascular fitness and body composition (higher lean to fatty weight ratio)
- Weight training to improve muscle strength and endurance
- Stretching to improve flexibility
- Proper nutrition to improve your health and body composition
- Anti-stress activity to keep your fitness program from driving you around the bend

A solid fitness program will usually lead to stress reduction, but it's an excellent idea to include an activity such as yoga or meditation which will specifically address stress.

Hint

The next few chapters will offer a more in-depth look at each of the components.

Chapter 5

Stop the Treadmill:
I Want to Get Off

WHAT IS CARDIOVASCULAR FITNESS?

Cardiovascular fitness, simply put, means that you have a healthy heart and blood vessels. A well-conditioned heart can pump more blood with each beat and get the same amount of work done with less effort, which is the same basic principle as using an industrial strength vacuum to clean your house instead of a Dustbuster.

AEROBIC EXERCISE

In order to attain cardiovascular fitness, aside from eating right, you've got to do some type of aerobic exercise. I like to think of this as sustained physical activity that raises your heart rate, causes you to sweat like a pig (not to be confused with glow), makes you tired and sore, and is nowhere near as much fun as sex. But like sex, unless you're very good at it and extremely self-conscious, you'll probably look stupid while you're doing it.

For instance, on a bicycle or in bed, never let your head drop all the way forward because your face will sag toward the ground. Most women over forty are acutely aware of this phenomenon, but my husband didn't have a clue as to what I was talking about until I had him bend his head over and look in a mirror. He was so shocked, he didn't speak to me for days. Like a lot of men, he also makes funny faces when he's working out and doesn't care if his sneakers are the correct shade to go with his gym shorts (two pitfalls that can so easily be avoided).

Aerobic activity involves the exhaustion and replenishment of the oxygen supply carried by the blood during continuous exercise of large muscle groups. A physically fit body is able to provide greater quantities of oxygen to the muscles. The muscles themselves exhibit certain changes which make them better able to utilize the oxygen. The end result is an even greater increase in strength, energy, and endurance. In other words, you'll be able to run around the block without heart palpitations, shortness of breath, muscle cramps, and the desire to lay down in the path of an oncoming car.

The concept of aerobic exercise may not turn you on too much because it's a lot of time and effort for something that's more of an internal benefit. But after forty, you really don't have a choice, unless, of course, you're interested in having high blood pressure and heart attacks.

On the bright side, it burns calories. Some experts even believe that aerobic activity will increase your **basal metabolic rate**, the level of energy required to perform vital functions such as respiration and repair, for several hours after you finish exercising, allowing you to continue burning extra calories. Some experts refute this, but who cares what they think?

Done long enough and at the right intensity, aerobic activity burns fat as well as calories. However, contrary to what you may have heard, "spot reducing" is a myth. You can tone the muscles in a particular area of your body but, unfair as it may seem, you can't select the areas of fat that you'd like to disappear first. Fat loss is a gradual, overall process.

Personally, I'll never understand why something which arrives at the hips and thighs takes off from a completely different location. This shoots a big hole in my theory that God is a woman because She would never do anything so perverse. On the other hand, this could be a god with a very sick sense of humor, or perhaps a god who worked out this section of the divine plan while she had a severe case of PMS.

EFFECTIVE AEROBICS WITHIN YOUR TRAINING ZONE

The trick to doing an effective aerobic workout is to find the pace that will burn fat and improve your cardiovascular system without overtaxing it. The following are a few different methods for determining your training zone.

Finding Your Pulse Rate. If you don't have a pulse monitor, use your middle and index fingers to locate the pulse at the base of your wrist or at the side of your neck near the Adam's apple. Count the number of beats in six seconds and then multiply by ten to calculate your heart rate in beats per minute.

Target Heart Rate Formula

Using this method, find your target heart rate zone and then exercise within that range by manually checking your pulse or by using an inexpensive pulse monitor. Many of the newer bikes and stair climbing machines have monitors built in.

Here's the basic formula:

a. Find your approximate maximum heart rate.
   220 − age = maximum heart rate (your real age, not the one you tell people who are tacky enough to ask)
b. Find your lower heart rate limit for aerobic exercise.
   Maximum heart rate x .60 = lower limit
c. Find your upper heart rate limit.
   Maximum heart rate x .80 = upper limit
d. Your target heart rate zone is within your upper and lower limits.

EXAMPLE

If you are 50 years old:
220 − 50 = 170
170 x .60 = 102
170 x .80 = 136

Your target heart rate is between 102 and 136 beats per minute.

These figures are only a conservative guideline and may vary by about ten percent according to your level of fitness.

Warning

This formula was designed for asymptomatic, physically active people without coronary artery disease risk factors or diagnosed disease. If you have any of these problems, were previously inert, or are taking medication, it's important to get medical clearance before you begin any exercise program. Actually, when you're over forty, it's not a bad idea to get medical clearance before you get out of bed in the morning.

The Borg Method

Gunnar Borg, a Swedish psychologist, introduced the ratings of perceived exertion (RPE) or Borg Scale, another method for determining if you're working at the appropriate intensity. During stress tests on treadmills, patients consult a chart and select a number that reflects the way they're feeling at any given moment.

The RPE Scale is numbered vertically from six to twenty, a six reflecting a restful state with virtually no exertion and a twenty reflecting the hardest possible workout. Descriptive terms, such as "very, very light" at seven to "very, very hard" at nineteen, simplify the procedure. Since most patients are able to give consistent RPE values for a variety of work intensities, this means that they can replicate the results of their treadmill tests when they exercise.

In learning how you feel when your heart is beating at, say, seventy per cent of maximum on the treadmill, you'll become more in tune with your body. Eventually you'll know instinctively how hard you're training and will be able to exercise at a pace that feels right.

The Morrow Scale

The Morrow Scale, named after an American exercise princess, is less scientific than Borg's but makes it very easy to gauge exertion. The basic principle is that if you have enough breath in you to do a lot of complaining while you're working out, you don't need a chart or a formula to tell you that you're doing something right. It indicates that you're breathing normally, as opposed to hyperventilating, and won't have to embarrass yourself by putting a paper bag over your face. (That is how they slow down breathing isn't it?)

As an added benefit, this method also assures you that although you're working hard and making some sacrifices, you're not developing a martyr complex, a very unpleasant side effect of too much exercise. On the other hand, if you want to double check to be sure that you're pushing yourself hard enough, all you have to do is stop complaining long enough to take your pulse. (See target heart rate formula.)

The Sweat Method

Sweat is another handy yardstick to let you know if you're putting out enough effort. When your sweat band turns from a fashion accessory to a necessity, you're on the right track. However, if you start sweating so much that people around you begin ducking for cover or skidding on the floor, you can turn it down just a touch.

White leotards are not a smart choice when you're doing aerobic exercise unless you're single or very desperate.

A WORD ABOUT INTENSITY

If you have a choice of working at a very high intensity for a short time or a low to moderate intensity for a longer period, opt for the latter. You'll not only achieve aerobic fitness, but will also have fewer medical problems and injuries, burn more fat, and be more likely to stick with it. If for some reason you have to work at a lower pace or intensity than is recommended, increase the length of your workouts or the number of sessions per week.

THE THREE STAGES OF AN AEROBIC WORKOUT

An average aerobic workout has three distinct physical and psychological phases.

Phase I—The Warm-up

a.k.a. "I'm never going to be able to do this."

You may have heard or discovered for yourself that the first ten minutes of an aerobic workout (running, biking, swimming, etc.) are brutal. This is true. In the first place, your body hasn't warmed up. In the second place, your **endorphins**, natural pain suppressants released by the brain when certain nerves are stimulated, haven't kicked in, and in the third place, you can't believe how much you have left to do. When you've only been running for twenty seconds, even twenty minutes seems like an eternity.

The release of endorphins is like taking drugs, only safer and more cost effective. Don't be fooled when you see women who seem to be having the time of their lives working out. It's just that they have more endorphins than you do. The same goes for people who play rugby or

pole vault. They'd never do those things if they knew how bad they really felt.

To get through this initial stage, warm up slowly, letting your heart rate and breathing increase gradually. Try distracting yourself until you get into a more comfortable groove.

Warning

Distracting yourself is much more feasible if you're doing an individual activity. If you distract yourself too much in a group, you'll get lost. You won't have a clue as to what everyone else is doing, and they'll probably be pointing at you and laughing.

If, however, you're one of those women who enjoy the music and motivation of an aerobics class but prefer to do your own thing—like hopping around in front of the mirror and chanting as if trying to get in touch with the exercise gods—more power to you. I really don't have a problem with this, although I like to do it in the privacy of my own home

Phase II—The Main Workout
a.k.a. "Damn, I'm good."

This is the "heart" of your workout. You've gotten over your initial resistance, your muscles have warmed up, and you're in your training zone. With any luck, your endorphins have also kicked in so you're feeling no pain. You can almost sense your heart getting stronger and the fat melting away. As you get more into shape and your endurance improves, you'll be able to extend or intensify this portion.

Phase III—The Cool Down
a.k.a. "Thank God it's almost over."

No matter how terrific you're feeling during a workout, eventually there'll come a point when your body will say "That's it. I've had enough." Before you experience lightheadedness, dizziness, shortness of breath, or muscle fatigue, it's time to cool down. Slow your pace so that your breathing returns to normal and your heart rate drops to 110 beats per minute or below. The cool down is generally very satisfying unless you've gotten overly compulsive and wish you had the stamina to continue for another hour or two. Your more common reaction will be, "Yes, yes, I'm done. Time to eat."

CARDIOVASCULAR BENEFITS

If you need some instant inspiration, here's a handy list of cardiovascular benefits. Memorize it and recite it to yourself as you're trying to zip up those pants that fit just last week, or as you're catching your breath after going out to get the mail:

- Decreased body fat
- Lower blood pressure
- Stronger heart
- Increased energy and endurance
- Increased basal metabolic rate
- New friends
- Condescending attitude toward lazy people
- Legitimate excuse to wear spandex and outrageous colors

Chapter 6

Aerobic Alternatives:
Pick Your Poison

DON'T JUST STAND THERE, DO SOMETHING!

There are so many different forms of aerobic exercise, that unless you're one of the ten laziest women on the face of the earth, you should be able to find something that appeals to you. Enjoyment is a key factor because if you don't like what you're doing, you'll never stick with it. (You know, like with sex.)

I thought that I could offer you some help in making your selection by sharing my experiences, both positive and negative, with various forms of exercise. Give them a try. If they don't work for you, consider other options such as swimming, skating, or dancing. The important point is not what you do, but that you do something!

Some of the following activities, such as jogging, are high-impact, sometimes called "hard." This means that they are more forceful and involve jumping or pounding movements which put more stress on your body. If done too often or for too long, these activities may become very uncomfortable.

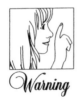

High impact activities may necessitate more bathroom breaks (especially if you've had kids).

Warning

Low-impact or "soft" workouts, such as cycling and walking, are usually non-jarring and therefore easier on the joints and on the bladder. Although low-impact exercise may not be as intense, if done properly and for an adequate duration, it will provide an excellent workout.

CHOICES

JOGGING

I don't jog, not that I have anything against it. It's just that I have an irrational fear that jogging will cause my uterus to fall out. This isn't necessarily a bad thing, especially if it's time for it to go, but I feel it's a bit too personal to experience in public. I can't imagine having to stop and pick it up, or even worse, having a stranger tap me on the shoulder and say, "Excuse me, ma'am, I believe you dropped this."

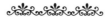

Personal Anecdote: "To Jog or Not to Jog"

Several years ago, I gave jogging a serious try. I was at a track sprinting with my kids when I suddenly thought that running might not be a bad idea. I didn't realize how much difference there would be between running short, fast races for fun and jogging long distances at a moderate pace for conditioning. In my naiveté, I bought an expensive pair of running shoes and headed back to the track, bragging to anyone who'd listen about how I was going to take the jogging world by storm.

My effort was doomed from the first lap, which, by the way, felt nothing like sprinting. A voice inside my head kept repeating, "I hate this. I hate this." Runners I'd spoken to had advised me to get into a rhythm, but I don't think that this was the rhythm they had in mind.

Not wanting to give up too easily, especially since I had the shoes, I moved over to a rolling cross-country course, hoping that the change in scenery would do the trick. The course, which looped through the agricultural school of a local community college and was populated with sheep, cattle, and pigs, turned out to be too challenging for my taste. Not only did I have to contend with the hills, but I had to be constantly on the alert not to step in something or cause a stampede.

Still not ready to quit, I tried getting my dog to run with me because I'd heard that dogs love to run. (Has anyone ever asked them?) Contrary to what I'd expected, my dog picked up on my attitude, hated jogging more than I did, and hid in the closet whenever she'd see me put on the shoes.

I'll share the two words that rescued me from jogging—"rainy season." Acting like it was a tremendous sacrifice, I put my running on hold and prayed that by the time the sun came out again no one would remember my previous boasts.

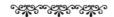

Pointers for Joggers

Although my experience was not very positive, sensible jogging can provide a great cardiovascular workout. Runners I've spoken to claim that it's also very relaxing and helps them think more clearly, making it easier to deal with other aspects of their lives. Some even say that they feel euphoric when they run.

Just be sure to play it safe so that you don't loosen any random body parts, put excessive strain on your joints and heart, or develop extra wrinkles (another of my theories). Follow these simple guidelines:

1. Get a decent pair of well-fitting running shoes that will cushion your feet and give you essential support.
2. Wear a jogging bra or some other form of cruel and unusual underwear.
3. Avoid running on concrete or other hard, unyielding surfaces, opting instead for softer ground or tracks, which will absorb some of the impact.
4. Try to run softly and quietly, staying light on your feet.
5. Find a knowledgeable person to show you how to run properly.
6. Check into community service programs, track clubs, and local Y's to find classes for mature but inexperienced runners. By joining a group, you'll be able to learn proper form and technique, monitor your progress, and meet other people who'll inspire you, motivate you, or, as in my case, out-complain you.

STAIRCLIMBING

During my brief stint at the stadium track, I'd occasionally see people walking or running up and down the bleacher steps. For awhile I kept my distance, assuming they were either taking part in a scientific study on insanity or were inmates from a minimum security prison. Eventually, my curiosity got the best of me. I decided to give the stairs a try.

After going up and down twice, despite moving very slowly for fear that I'd trip and break my neck, I was gasping for air. But much to my shock—I liked it. It was probably due to the required level of concentration, which didn't leave me much time to think about what I was doing, and to the periodic reinforcement of reaching the top. Each time

I climbed the last step, I could hear the theme music from *Rocky* as I'd leap in the air and shake my fists.

This type of exercise isn't for everyone, but if you're in outstanding condition and looking for a challenge, a more strenuous change of pace, or a way to shape up your rear end, it's an option.

Keep that last benefit in mind the next time you have your finger on an elevator call button. The elevator may be quicker and easier, but stairs will do more for your body.

Hint

Pointers for Stairclimbers
1. Find wooden steps which have some give to them, will absorb the impact, and be less jarring.
2. When you go up the steps, strive to lift your legs high so that you really work your quadriceps, glutes and hamstrings.
3. When you descend, be sure to walk, not run, so that you don't destroy your knees.
4. If you have any knee problems whatsoever, forget stairclimbing.
5. Try to keep moving, even when you get tired, so that your heart rate stays elevated. Instead of flopping down on the ground, walk around on a flat surface until you recoup your energy.
6. Stay slow and steady. Concentrate on what you're doing.

WALKING
An alternative to running and stairclimbing is walking. It's not as demanding but is certainly less risky. I'm referring to plain old fitness walking, sometimes called power walking or striding, in which you move with a normal gait at a faster than normal speed for a specified period of time. Contrary to what you may have seen, it's not necessary to wear a long dress with tennis shoes, nor carry shopping bags when you do this.

Let me clarify that when I refer to power walking I'm not alluding to racewalking, in which the participants strut down the street like crazed ducks, going as fast as they possibly can. If you want to get into that you're on your own. I could never recommend anything which looks so goofy and also involves unnatural movements that may be hard on your joints.

Advantages of Walking

Walking is a perfect form of exercise because it's safe, it's easy, it's low-impact, it requires no special equipment, and it allows you to keep up a fairly in-depth conversation with yourself or with a companion. A walking program is especially well-suited to older women or to women who have been inactive or incapacitated.

Another plus of walking is that you can do it anywhere. You can walk at the beach and get some extra resistance from the sand, around a track, along the street, or even in shopping malls early in the morning.

Many experts agree that a brisk twenty to thirty minute walk, three to five times per week, will condition your body about as well as any other aerobic activity. In addition, a reasonable estimate would be that a woman walking at a comfortable (not slow) pace could burn up to three hundred calories in an hour.

Walking Pointers

1. With cardiovascular guidelines for intensity and duration in mind, walk at a pace that suits your fitness level. To check yourself, walk for ten minutes, find your heart rate, and see if you're in your training zone.
2. Even though you've been walking for most of your life, when you're doing it as serious exercise, you must be conscious of your form. Walk erect but relaxed, arms swinging freely and naturally, knees slightly bent. Instead of landing flat-footed, roll forward from the front of your heels through the balls of your feet.
3. Wear comfortable, well-fitting shoes with adequate cushioning and support.
4. Walking research indicates that 3.0 to 3.5 mph is an average pace, 3.75 to 4 mph is considered brisk, and 5.0 mph or more is for very well-conditioned walkers. Keep in mind that these figures are for striding or power walking, not for strolling. Your pace on a treadmill may also be slower, especially if you have a short stride.

You can safely assume that if your clothes are out of style by the time you get around the block, you're going too slow.

Hint

Walking with Weights

After you've been on a walking program for awhile and have improved your fitness level to the point that you can maintain a high intensity workout within your training zone, you can add light weights to your routine. For starters, go back to an easier walk, but this time carry a half pound weight in each hand. As you become better conditioned, increase the weights in half pound increments until you reach a maximum of two pounds in each hand. Once you get used to the weights, you can do simple arm routines with them similar to the ones they do in aerobics. This may look silly, but it still won't look as silly as racewalking.

Don't use ankle weights when walking because they'll dramatically increase the impact stress on your feet, legs, knee and hip joints.

Warning

AEROBICS CLASSES

Aerobics classes, still one of the most popular forms of exercise, have been refined and expanded over the years. They now come disguised in so many different sizes and shapes, even women who've sworn off aerobics don't realize that they're still doing them. From high-impact to low-impact, from dancercise to boxercise, there's something for everyone. Can it be long before eatercise and shoppercise are sweeping the country?

❦❦❦

Personal Anecdote: Aerobics "Barbie"

I can remember my first aerobics class as if it was yesterday. Deep down inside, I knew it wasn't for me because I'm not overly coordinated and because I like to be in control of my workouts. (If I want someone telling me what to do, I can give my unlisted number to my kids.) Nevertheless, I was talked into it by the locker room regulars who carried on about the energy level, the fun, the music, and the male instructors in tight shorts.

I donned my leotard, tights, fashionable workout shoes, sweat band, wrist bands, and pseudo-perky attitude, then strutted into the room. Having seen the no-sweat aerobics groupies who'd walk out at the end of an hour looking exactly like they had when they'd walked in—cool, calm, hair and make-up perfect—I figured it couldn't be all that difficult.

Then the teacher bounced in the door! Much to my dismay, instead of a stud in shorts, it was "Aerobics Barbie," young, gorgeous, athletic, and depressingly peppy. She couldn't even spell cellulite, let alone find any on her body. No wonder she couldn't stop smiling.

The first part of the class wasn't unpleasant—a light warm-up and some gentle stretching. Just as I began to wonder why I'd had any reservations, "Barbie" picked up the tempo and went for blood. The faster she went, the more intricate the movements became. She was a hopeless show-off who performed fancy footwork as her right arm did one thing and her left arm did something totally unrelated. She whipped the class into a frenzy, encouraging us to yell as if we were at a revival meeting. As I tried to do a reasonable facsimile of what most of the others were doing, I kept asking myself, "Why didn't I have someone page me out of here at a pre-arranged time?"

After what seemed like hours of running and jumping, the music slowed down and everyone grabbed mats and sprawled out on the floor. Assuming it was time for a well-deserved nap, I was about to join them when "Barbie" gleefully announced that we were going to do abdominals and other muscle isolation exercises. Since I was down low,

46

I tried to slither out of the room, but a couple of self-appointed aerobics commandos caught me and dragged me back.

The music picked up again and we were forced to do so many crunches and sit-ups, I thought I'd lose my lunch. These were followed by an excruciating series of leg lifts. When the instructor chirped that we were about to do "dog at the fire hydrant," I thought "That's it, I'm outta here." I managed to make it to the end of the hour by fantasizing about "Barbie" getting old and fat.

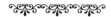

Aerobics Pointers

1. The instructor can make or break a class so do some checking before you sign up. Ask around or observe a few sessions. Look for a knowledgeable, certified instructor whose style and personality are compatible with your own.
2. Select a class that's appropriate for your level of ability whether it's beginning, advanced, or intermediate.
3. Consider low-impact instead of the more traditional high impact classes. The toll on your body will be a lot less.
4. Work at your own pace. Don't try to keep up with everyone else around you.
5. Remember, no matter how lost you may feel in a class, eventually the routines will get so familiar that you'll stop stepping on your own feet and smacking other people with your arms.
6. Don't be fooled by the warm-up. It's designed to lull you into a false sense of security before the music changes and the instructor tries to make you beg for mercy.
7. Fake it by smiling and yelling "whoopee." Everyone will think you've gotten into the spirit and will stop picking on you.

Alternative Aerobics Classes

Now that you're no longer obligated to take the traditional high-impact classes, consider some of the other options.

Low-impact Step Classes. In step classes, a small set of adjustable stairs is integrated into the routines. You begin by using one step board. As you progress, you can increase the difficulty by adding step risers. This is a non-jarring way to get extra leg workout and to challenge yourself within the structure of a class.

Water Aerobics. Water aerobics classes, taught in a pool, are especially beneficial for older women and for women with arthritis. The water acts as a cushion, making the movements safer and more comfortable, while at the same time providing additional resistance. The next time you're at a pool, wade in until the water is waist high. Then try to walk quickly or run over to the wall. You'll feel exactly how the water resistance works.

Wear a one-piece bathing suit or you may end up flashing everyone in the pool. If the thought of putting on a bathing suit is too traumatic, no matter how many pieces it comes in, wear a T-shirt and a pair of shorts with a secure waist. Aside from offering additional coverage, the extra fabric will add resistance.

Rubber Band Aerobics. These classes incorporate large sturdy rubber bands or rubber tubing into the routines. During repeated movements, the intensity of the exercise is increased by pulling against the muscles with the rubber band. The added resistance simulates working with light weights or with a partner. Some bodybuilders use surgical tubing to get their muscles pumped up at competitions, especially when there are no available free weights.

If you have any apprehension about the rubber band snapping on you, don't bother with these classes. You won't be able to concentrate.

STATIONARY EQUIPMENT

Cardiovascular equipment (stationary bikes, treadmills, skiers, stairclimbers, etc.) offers a viable workout alternative. As with every form of exercise, there are advantages and disadvantages.

Advantages

- You're in control, regulating the length and intensity of the workout.
- You can use them whenever the mood strikes
- There's no peer pressure.
- There are no bossy instructors telling you what to do.

Disadvantages

- Machines are boring.
- You have to be self-motivated and self-disciplined.
- You must have the patience, determination, and imagination to walk, row, or cycle for an extended period while going nowhere.

Warning

Stairclimbing machines offer similar benefits to step walking without the risks, however, two common mistakes undermine their effectiveness.

> *1. Avoid putting so much pressure on your arms that your feet are practically dangling in the air.*
> *2. Avoid taking such teeny steps that the only things getting a workout are the soles of your shoes. Instead, hold on lightly for balance and security and take large enough steps that your legs and rear end get in on the action.*

Breaking the Monotony

An effective way to break the tedium of the machines is to split your routine into two or three parts. Try rowing for fifteen minutes, cycling for fifteen more, and ending with a ten minute walk on the treadmill. This method gives you the added advantage of working different muscle groups.

Many costlier machines attempt to stimulate you by having you race against miniature figures on a computer screen. The rower, for example, will display your boat and another one, constantly informing you how many boat lengths ahead or behind you are, as if you really care.

If for some unexplainable reason you enjoy that sort of harassment, more power to you, but nine out of ten women whom I've surveyed hate it. Men, on the other hand, love it. It's some sort of hormonal imbalance so they really can't help themselves. They seem to get a testosterone rush out of beating the other boat. In my experience, staying on the machines is challenging enough without having to compete with an imaginary opponent. Besides, you should always cover the screen with a towel in order to block out the digital time readout. (More about that under motivation.)

Don't wear a thong leotard if you're going to be seated on stationary equipment unless you have a fondness for rug burns.

Warning

Purchasing Home Equipment

If you can afford the luxury of purchasing equipment for your home (it will save you time and health club fees) here are some other points to consider:

1. Although there's a wide price range for each type of machine, you generally get what you pay for and none of them are inexpensive enough to serve as coat racks or oversized dust collectors.

2. Before you purchase a piece of equipment, insist on ample time to try it out, even if you have to go to a club to do so. Five minutes on a bike is not a sufficient test run. Be sure that the machine is sturdy, comfortable, and that you like using it.

3. Check into maintenance, repair, and warranty procedures. See if parts and service are local or if there's a main number to call.

4. Be sure that you have adequate space for the machine.

5. Find out if it can be adjusted to fit your body or anyone else's who may be using it.

6. See if you can change the resistance while you're on it. Check if

it has convenient gauges, such as a speedometer or heart monitor.

7. Think about purchasing used equipment. Many people buy machines, use them once or twice, then can't unload them fast enough. Check market and health club bulletin boards for bargains or look in your local recycler.

8. Inquire about renting equipment before you buy. Some stores offer this option.

Triathlons

I'm including this topic for the truly desperate women who will stop at nothing to get in shape and for those of you who may be desperate enough to let them talk you into it.

Triathlons are athletic contests in which you swim, bike, and run for specified distances. I have no quarrel with them if done on a very limited scale (although I can't imagine why you'd want to crawl out of the water looking like a drowned rat and jump on a bike). But the ones that involve long distances completely baffle me. It had to be a sick mind that came up with the concept of swimming over two miles, pedaling a hundred more on a bike, and then, just for laughs, running a marathon.

Whenever I meet women who're involved in full length triathlons, I have the urge to keep questioning them until I can understand their motivation. It's like trying to fathom what goes on in the mind of a serial killer—a morbid fascination with alien behavior.

When a woman at the gym excitedly informed me that she'd won the lottery for the Ironman (the big daddy of triathlons), I said, "That's great, now you don't have to go." She stared at me as if I was crazy and explained that so many people wanted to sign up, that a lottery was held to select the entrants. Funny, I'd always assumed that they blackmailed people into participating.

If you feel that you must do a triathlon in this lifetime or die an unhappy woman, I strongly urge you to consider the mini versions. Mini-triathlons substantially decrease the mileage on each segment, enabling you to experience the thrill of competition without the agony of self-abuse. They also allow you to derive the benefits of cross-training without going to detrimental extremes.

MARTIAL ARTS

The martial arts offer a "kick butt" workout that allows you to release your aggression while getting in shape and learning how to defend yourself. Whether feisty or fainthearted, you can train to develop your protective instincts as you condition your body.

⸙⸙⸙

PERSONAL ANECDOTE: "THE KARATE OLD PERSON"

As with so many activities, I became involved in martial arts before I had a chance to realize what I was doing. I was innocently picking up dry cleaning, when a woman I'd known for years through the exercise circuit came running up to me exclaiming, "I found a new class you have to try. Karate." I replied, "Karate? Uniforms, discipline, fighting. Are you kidding?" But when I peeked in the window of the studio next door, I was so intrigued by what I saw that I agreed to stop back the next morning to observe the women only class.

The following day, I walked into the school and was about to take a seat in the back of the room, when the instructor— barefoot, dressed in white pajamas with a black belt—approached me, bowed and introduced himself. Not sure what to do, I stood up, bowed back, and told him that I was looking forward to watching the class. He then informed (yes, informed) me that I'd be participating.

Not wanting to cause a scene, and intimidated by the unfamiliarity of the situation and the mean look on his face, I removed my shoes and bowed my way onto the exercise mat. For the next hour, I tried to hide behind the other women as we went through formal routines of conditioning, stretching, kicking and punching. No one spoke unless spoken to by the instructor, but there was a whole lot of yelling, grunting, and "yes, sirring" going on. Frankly, I was stunned because I knew some of these women and had never seen them behave like this. They didn't even know the meaning of obedience and generally couldn't stop talking long enough to get their teeth cleaned.

We did exercises to strengthen and stretch the muscles. We toughened our hands and feet by pounding on special pads (great for frustration).

We practiced on imaginary opponents, targets, punching bags, and even on each other. We learned stances (certain ways to stand), blocking techniques to use if anyone tried to attack us, as well as ways to attack.

Although I was initially too embarrassed to make a sound, after awhile I began shouting like a woman who's just had her legs waxed for the first time. The main reason was that the instructor made me do push-ups every time I refused to yell. I later learned that the sound, a loud "kiah" (or whatever works for you), puts more force in your movement, helps with breathing, and intimidates an opponent.

At the close of that first class, I bowed my way out of the studio, stumbled to my car, drove home and fell asleep for three hours. The next day, despite all of my previous exercising, brand-new parts of my body—parts that I hadn't even known existed— were asking, "What have you done to us this time?" I knew I was on to something.

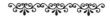

Different Styles of Martial Arts

Even within karate, which is one of several Oriental forms of unarmed combat, there are variations. Most styles use the same basic skills, but with different emphasis and technique. For instance, tae kwon do, Korean karate, stresses kicking and hard, powerful movements. Kung fu, which is Chinese, uses more flowing, circular motion. Tai chi, another Chinese form, is particularly well-suited for older women because it excludes extreme movements and instead emphasizes balance, coordination, and effortlessness. There are women in their eighties and nineties who practice tai chi. If you're better at yelling and confrontation than at balance and coordination, I'd suggest the more aggressive varieties. Attitude can cover up a multitude of mistakes.

Advantages and Disadvantages

Most karate students advance through ranks of achievement, designated by belts of different colors. Beginners wear white, experts wear black, with various colors in between. Promotions are earned by testing before a group of judges, demonstrating that you've mastered the skills which are the prerequisites for the next rank.

Despite the fact that the belt system offers increasingly difficult motivational goals and periodic reinforcement, I have a couple of issues with it. In the first place, it's somewhat stressful and in the second, call me shallow, but I don't like the colors of the belts. Yellow and orange are two of the most common, and I never wear those shades.

While I'm being shallow, I may as well elaborate on my feelings about the uniforms. I'm sure you've seen them—baggy, white cotton pants with an unflattering, uncomfortable white jacket that makes it difficult to move and adds about ten pounds to your appearance. To be fair, the pants do prevent anyone from seeing your thighs jiggle when you kick.

On a more positive note, the study of martial arts improves your awareness and your ability to focus. It also develops confidence and self-assurance. I was very impressed by the changes I observed in other women after they'd been studying for only a few months. Even those who were normally quite timid became more assertive and aggressive. As a matter of fact, some of them became downright cocky.

If practiced with caution, the martial arts afford an exciting change of pace from the monotony of established routines. There's something to be said for a regimen that strengthens you, stretches you, improves your cardiovascular system, increases your awareness and skill, and at the same time encourages you to tear the heart out of anyone who even looks at you funny.

HIKING

PERSONAL ANECDOTE: "AH, WILDERNESS"

In high school, I was voted "least likely to ever go hiking." I was very flattered because even though I'd never actually met any female hikers, I had a definite image in mind. They were overgrown Girl Scouts who carried backpacks, wore clunky tan boots, unattractive khaki shorts and blouses, and had Swiss army knives hanging from their belts.

With this picture in mind, when a couple of acquaintances from the gym asked if I'd like to go hiking with them, I was about to blurt out, "You must be joking!" when I realized that they both shaved their legs and wore makeup when they worked out. Of course, they were men, but they were quite tasteful nonetheless. I'm kidding, it was two women and since neither fit my preconceptions about hikers, I agreed to join them the next day.

We parked on a street not five minutes from my house, walked down a slight incline, and were suddenly out in the country. Even having lived in the neighborhood for fifteen years, I'd never realized that I was so close to nature—a creek, tree covered hills, wild flowers, birds, bugs. I'd heard people talk about the area from time to time. I'd even seen the mountains from a distance, but I'd never entertained the thought of actually going there and getting dirty.

We set off down a fire road that paralleled the creek, then gently ribboned its way to the top of a small mountain. From there we took a narrow but picturesque trail that brought us up even higher. After oohing and aahing over the spectacular view, we retraced our steps and headed back to the cars. Entranced by the experience, I couldn't wait to go again. I even agreed to buy hiking boots.

For our next trek, we met at the same spot and started down the same gentle hill. Then everything changed. My intrepid guides decided that instead of the fire road, which was for wimps, we should try a "real" trail up the side of the mountain. Being a newborn nature woman ready to conquer all, also being an idiot, I said, "sure" and followed along.

Stumbling through rocks and underbrush, we located a trail. I use the term loosely because I don't think anyone had been on it since the pioneers. It was so steep and narrow that once we started the climb, all I ever saw was the dirt under my nose. Toward the top, the trail was even more precipitous. We practically crawled the last few hundred feet. To make matters worse, insects were dive bombing our heads and lizards were dashing across our feet.

Wiping the sweat out of our eyes long enough to glance at the view, we began our descent on a trail that was not only steep, but covered with loose, slippery gravel. I was sure that at any moment I was going to plunge over the side and disappear. I had a terrible vision of having to be rescued, the rescue being shown on the news, and hundreds of people asking, "How could this middle-aged woman be dumb enough to get herself into this situation and be wearing such ugly shoes?"

When we finally made it back to the cars, I was drained. I also thought I was cured of hiking, but the experience must have tapped into the vein of insanity that runs in my family because a few days later there I was again, standing at the base of a mountain, ready for more.

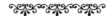

To Hike or Not to Hike

If you love the outdoors, hiking may be just the thing for you. This is especially true if you reside in a temperate climate which is conducive to "exercise alfresco." Living in an area with varied terrain makes it even better, but you may not realize what's available to you until you start exploring.

From a strictly physical standpoint, hiking develops your stamina and endurance while at the same time strengthening your muscles. Trekking up and down hills works your quadriceps, hamstrings, glutes (butt muscles), and calves. In very rugged areas your upper body may also get a workout as you grab on to roots and branches to keep from sliding into oblivion.

You just have to be judicious, not going further than you can handle or on trails that are too rough for your level of experience. You should also pay particular attention to your knees and back to be sure that they're not being overtaxed.

Aside from conditioning, the allure of hiking is that it affords the opportunity for getting away from it all. You can leave your troubles behind and put your responsibilities on hold. Out in the wild, there are no televisions, radios, fax machines, or telephones—well, almost no telephones. One of my friends brings her cellular along, and we spend half the time wondering why no one is calling us.

Furthermore, hiking gives you an uncanny knack for solving the problems of the world. I don't know whether it's due to being in touch with nature or out of touch with reality, but you'll suddenly find yourself able to handle anything from dysfunctional families to job hassles to international affairs. For instance, one afternoon, while fighting off heatstroke because we hadn't believed the weatherman who'd predicted hundred degree temperature, we got on the topic of global warming. It only took us a few minutes to figure out that the hole in the ozone layer was almost single-handedly being caused by our mutual hairdresser and his cavalier use of cans of hair spray with fluorocarbon propellants.

When not solving problems, you'll probably find yourself discussing food. You can work up quite an appetite while hiking. Since there are no restaurants out in the wilderness (a regrettable condition along with the lack of bathrooms), talk often turns to what you'd like to be eating, what you plan to eat when you finish, and what you should have eaten before you started out.

This is embarrassing to admit, but one afternoon I even caught myself sharing recipes with a companion who has almost as many excuses as I do for not cooking. We promised never to tell anyone about the incident, so I won't name names. I will only reveal that this is the same person with the cellular phone and that we got so hungry, we tried calling and ordering a large pizza but they wouldn't deliver without an address.

For those of you who are afraid that you're too old to hike, I've encountered many senior citizens on the trails who are in fabulous shape. I met a woman of about seventy, hiking by herself (which I don't recommend), wearing a large, heavy backpack. She informed me that she was practicing for her annual hike in the high Sierras, much rougher territory than I'd ever attempted. On another occasion, some friends and I hiked with a man whom we judged to be about sixty and could barely stay up with him. Imagine our surprise during a rest stop (our idea, not his) when we found out that he was seventy-six and had children who were twelve and fourteen! (I told you hiking improves stamina and endurance.)

Getting Started

If the idea of hiking appeals to you but you're not sure where to go or how to get started, check with the local Sierra Club, parkland conservancy groups, wilderness institutes, or camping stores. They can help you locate easy, moderate, and difficult trails. They may also offer guided hikes, a wonderful way to begin and to meet other people.

The Essentials

To hike comfortably and safely, you'll need certain essentials.

1. Since hiking is not a fashion statement, wear functional clothing. I'd suggest loose-fitting pants (long ones if you're going to be in brush), a couple of shirts to accommodate changes in temperature, and two pairs of socks, one to act as a liner. Naturally, in cool weather you should add a jacket, warm hat, and gloves. In warm weather, try a baseball hat to keep the sun off your hair and face, unless you want to wear one of those funky straw hats that makes you look as if you have a salad bowl on your head.

2. Like it or not, sturdy, well-fitting hiking boots are a must.

3. You'd be wise to bring sun block, insect repellent, a multi-purpose bandanna, and a basic first aid kit, if you can convince someone else to carry it for you. One of my friends also insists on bringing Krazy Glue in case she breaks a nail.

4. Dried fruit, granola, and other light snacks will provide needed energy.

5. Water is essential. Bring an amount that is appropriate for the climate and duration of the hike. Take a drink at least every twenty minutes whether or not you're thirsty.

If you want your water to stay cold, freeze a third of it, then fill up the rest of the bottle right before you leave. You can also purchase an insulated bag designed for carrying water bottles.

6. A compass is probably a good idea, although I have mixed feelings about it. I can't see the advantage of being able to find north if you're so confused that you have no idea which way you're attempting to go. Try trail maps if you can read them, or better yet, get a guide. It's too bad you can't buy a sense of direction.

Hint

Tying ribbons around trees is a practical variation on the Hansel and Gretel bread crumb technique for retracing your steps. It's also very festive, particularly around the holidays.

7. I hate to say it, but a Swiss army knife isn't a bad idea.
8. A decent sized fanny pack or small, lightweight backpack is handy for carrying all of your paraphernalia.

Hint

Camping or outdoor specialty stores are the best places to buy your equipment because they employ knowledgeable people who can provide useful advice. Keep in mind, though, that the people who work in these stores take themselves even more seriously than the people who work in health food stores. When a salesperson was showing me a fanny pack and I joked that it was perfect because it had compartments where I could carry makeup and hair spray, he snatched it out of my hands and refused to sell it to me.

Warning

Learn to identify the poisonous plants in your area. They usually contain an oil that's very irritating to your skin. If you come into contact with the oil, even by taking off your shoes after walking on the plant, you may end up with redness, blisters, and such horrendous itching that you won't know what not to scratch first. Wash with soap and cold water as soon as possible. In severe cases, consult a physician.

Ironically, some of these plants are quite pretty and make excellent gifts for people who make fun of you for hiking.

BIKING

(You'll probably be relieved to know that I don't have a personal anecdote on this topic.)

If you share the hiker's love for the freedom of outdoor exercise but need a bit more speed to hold your interest (and also enjoy sitting down), bike riding may be your answer. Bicycling offers a unique, non-polluting way to cover miles of countryside. It's an activity that you can enjoy into your eighties with none of the connective tissue damage that sometimes ravages runners.

Like hiking, biking can also be a very social activity, more pleasant and safer if you do it with other people. Through cycling stores or health clubs you can locate bicycling associations which organize rides for people of all different ages and abilities.

Cycling has gotten so popular in the last few years that millions of women are peddling, some strictly for fun and others for fitness. To accomplish the latter, you're going to have to work for the benefits. According to world renowned cyclist Greg LeMond, "Although bike riding is good, healthy exercise, the actual benefit derived from riding only a few miles a day at a purely recreational pace is only about equivalent to a slow, half-hour walk." If you prefer the slower pace, spend at least thirty to sixty minutes on your bike. Coasting with your feet off the pedals doesn't count.

Interestingly, many women of all ages who begin riding strictly for diversion find it so satisfying that they soon graduate to light touring, often traveling twenty to twenty-five miles a day. This is obviously much more conducive to getting in shape and losing fat than a few quick zips around the block.

Where to Cycle

Ideally, you should ride on clearly marked bike paths that wind through parks, along the beach, or in quiet residential neighborhoods. Even if you live in a busy urban area, you should be able to locate parks or specially designated trails for cycling. Try contacting the local department of parks and recreation for information. Sticking to these areas will not only prevent you from swallowing a variety of toxic exhaust fumes, but will also protect you from careless drivers or drivers with a grudge against bike riders.

If you have no other alternative besides city streets or are traveling in sparsely populated areas where you might encounter some major roads, be sure to ride to the right. Obey all traffic laws (a very important detail if you don't want to end up getting traffic tickets; not as important if you're interested in meeting a policeman). Finally, make yourself highly visible, using reflective strips on your clothing and helmet if necessary.

Some of the more daring riders are leaving the bike paths and streets and going off-road on rougher terrain, using sturdily built mountain bikes. Although this adventurous type of riding demands greater bike handling proficiency, it offers the chance for a rigorous workout while at the same time allowing you to appreciate the serenity of more secluded areas.

Equipment

The necessary gear for long-distance cycling or mountain biking is basically the same as for hiking, with the addition of a pump, tire patch, and simple tool kit. Oh yes, there is one major expense—a bicycle.

Before making a purchase, determine the type of riding that you'll be doing, whether it's primarily on streets and bike paths, off-road, or a little of each. There is a wide variety of available bicycles. One that is fine for easy outings may feel heavy and sluggish if you have to climb significant hills or decide to go long distances. Instead of looking forward to your next ride, you'll be looking forward to selling your bike for scrap metal.

Once you've narrowed down your selection, rent or borrow a few different models to see which you find most comfortable. You might also steal a bike from one of your children or grandchildren, who will have forgotten that she abandoned it in your garage until she spots you on it. Be strong. Don't give in when she tries to get it back.

Bikes, like stationary equipment, come in a wide price range, but again, you get what you pay for. Talk to other riders to find a dealer who's knowledgeable, has a broad selection, will make sure that your bike fits properly, will do repairs, and won't rip you off.

The Outfit

A helmet is a safety essential and in some areas a legal requirement. Although still not very chic, helmets are much lighter and more comfortable than they used to be. They're also your only protection if your head should hit the ground.

If you plan to do any serious riding, cycling shoes are a sensible purchase. They're lighter and less bulky than regular workout shoes, with leather or mesh tops that conform to your feet and let them breathe. They have special soles that grip the pedals more efficiently and absorb the force of the pedaling motion.

As for clothing, biking shorts are a must because they're almost cute enough to make up for the helmet. They're snug without being constricting, and they also have padded seats which prevent blisters on your backside. Best of all, they end about two inches above your knees so they cover your thighs.

If you have chubby knees, wear the longer length biking pants. They'll cover your knees and be more slenderizing.

Hint

For the top, cycling jerseys look very cool and offer sun protection, but you can save the expense by wearing a leotard or well-fitting shirt that won't flap around in the breeze. Nylon, foldable windbreakers are handy for accommodating sudden temperature changes.

When hiking or biking, before you hit the trail in warm weather, wash your hair and apply conditioner. Slick your hair back or braid it. When it's partially dry, put on a baseball hat or helmet and you're all set. The conditioner does its work while you're exercising. Simply wash it off in the shower when you get home. You'll have fabulous, healthy hair to go along with your fabulous, healthy body.

Hint

TIPS FOR AEROBIC SUCCESS

Whether you select one of the activities that I've included in this chapter or something entirely different, the guidelines (which are discussed in greater detail in later sections) remain the same.

1. Get started immediately because you're not getting any younger.
2. Break in gradually.
3. Warm up, stretch through your range of motion, exercise, then cool down. It's advisable to end your workout with a few minutes of more intense stretching. (See chapter on flexibility.)
4. Work within your training zone.
5. Aim for three to five workouts per week, lasting twenty to sixty minutes per session.
6. As you progress, increase the frequency, duration, or intensity of your workouts.

Chapter 7

Real Women Don't Iron: They Pump It

A BRIEF HISTORY OF WEIGHT TRAINING— MINE AND MILO'S

According to legend, the first known weight trainer was Milo of Crotona, a Greek wrestler in the ancient days when matches occasionally ended in death. Not really fancying that option, Milo determined to make himself the strongest and most physically fit wrestler in all of Greece. He began his training by slinging a young calf across his shoulders and walking around a stadium. As the calf grew older and heavier, Milo grew more powerful until he was acknowledged as the strongest man in the world.

Inadvertently, I began strength training in almost the identical manner. Wanting to be the strongest on my block and never being able to find a baby sitter, let alone a calf, I'd sling my daughter over my hips, around my neck, and onto my back. As I had more kids and as they grew heavier, I became tougher and sturdier. Just like Milo, I was applying the principle of progressive resistance exercise, better known as weight training. When I joined a gym, I simply switched to dumbbells, barbells, and other apparatus instead of using my children.

During my non-athletic childhood, I'd never heard of weight lifting or bodybuilding, so I was more surprised than anyone, except perhaps my entire extended family, when I began pumping iron on a regular basis. My grandmother submitted my name to *Ripley's Believe It or Not.* My cousins couldn't stop laughing long enough to congratulate me when I won my first bodybuilding competition, and my brother started calling me "Butch," which was probably preferable to what he'd been calling me before that.

WEIGHT LIFTING WILL NOT TURN YOU INTO A MAN

Many normally sensible women are afraid that if they so much as touch a weight machine, they'll turn into muscle-bound hulks with deep voices and bad attitudes. I had the same concerns when I first began lifting weights in a hard-core gym.

I used to watch in fascination as some of the brawnier women would bench press the combined weight of my family, curl barbells that most of the men couldn't lift off the rack, and squat with weights that would have killed a normal woman. Although I lived in fear of looking like them, especially when I realized that a few had beards and weren't even close to menopause, a part of me was a little envious of their progress and curious as to how they were getting such dramatic results.

When I summoned up the nerve to ask, they told me that it was due to excellent diet, high testosterone levels (I didn't even know women had testosterone), and superior training techniques, three elements which I was obviously lacking. I figured that two of them had to be sharing a cow for lunch to get that big.

One day, when I saw a syringe in the trash can, it finally hit me. These women were using steroids! Sure, they were training hard and eating well, but they were also getting help from the local pharmaceutical rep. In addition, they were getting hard faces, huge pimples on their backs, and very bad personalities, not the normal results of exercise. Although disgusted, in a strange sense I was relieved. I could train as hard as I wanted without turning into one of the guys. My husband was also quite comforted knowing that I wouldn't be fighting him for the after shave.

THE THREE MAIN BODY TYPES

Women with **mesomorphic,** naturally muscular physiques, are more apt to develop muscularity than **ectomorphic**, long and lean, or **endomorphic,** more fatty women. However, we're all a combination of body types and are also protected by our hormones from changing sex involuntarily. So don't be hesitant about developing your natural muscularity or you'll defeat the whole purpose of the workout. If worse comes to worse, you can always load up on estrogen.

REPS AND SETS

With weight lifting, as with every other aspect of fitness, you should determine your goals before you develop your routine. In this case, your training will be influenced by whether you want to substantially increase your size and strength or just tone up what you already have.

In order to understand the difference and to sound as if you know what you're talking about, here is some basic terminology:

- **Repetition:** ("rep" to the cool people) the cycle of lifting a weight and returning it to its starting place
- **Set:** a group of repetitions.

If you really want to impress people at parties you can also toss around the following words:

- **Buff:** very muscular
- **Ripped:** very lean with well-defined muscularity

TONING VS. BUILDING

If you're the average woman, desperately trying to tone up rather than turn into a female Arnold Schwarzenegger, your best bet is to select a weight that you can lift for ten to twelve reps. Once you can complete twelve reps, you can either rest briefly and do another set of the exercise, or increase the weight by about two and a half pounds at your next session. Eventually, you should be able to perform three sets of an exercise. If you get brave enough to go for a bit more size and strength, use heavier weights and do fewer reps in a set, perhaps only six or eight.

BREAKING DOWN THE BODY PARTS

For the purpose of weight training, the body is separated into six main parts with a few subdivisions. This may not be scientific, but it's a heck of a lot easier than trying to memorize every single muscle group when you can barely remember what you had for breakfast this morning.

These divisions are:

- Chest
- Back
- Shoulders
- Arms
  Biceps
  Triceps

- Legs
  Quadriceps
  Hamstrings
  Calves
  Gluteus muscles a.k.a. "your butt"
- Abdominals a.k.a. "abs"

In planning your routine, you have several options depending on your time, energy, and level of desperation. Ideally, you should do strength training two or three times a week, but if once is all you can manage, it's still better than nothing.

TRAINING COMBINATIONS

Full Body Circuit
If you can only make it once a week, you won't have much of a choice. You'll have to do it all, keeping your weights lighter and your number of sets down.

Upper-Lower
This is just what it sounds like. You do your upper body one time and lower body the next. An upper-lower routine is practical for twice-a-weekers. Abs and calves are done at each session.

Push-Pull
You work the pushing muscles (chest, shoulders, triceps) in one session and the pulling muscles (back, biceps) in another. Legs can be worked with either.

Random
You can make up a routine that you like. For instance, arms and legs one day, chest, back, and shoulders another.

Essentially, how you choose to combine muscle groups is not as important as getting the job done. Find a routine that works for you, stop talking about it, and do it.

BASIC EXERCISES THAT WORK AT ANY AGE

If you don't have dumbbells, try filling small, plastic bottles with sand or water. Vary the resistance by adding or subtracting sand or water.

Hint

Over the years, I've experimented with all sorts of exercises for each muscle group, some effective and some so ridiculous that I hope no one ever finds out about them. Although I still try out new techniques, I usually find myself gravitating back to the basics. Perhaps this is a perfect example of that saying about old dogs and new tricks.

The following are suggested exercises for old dogs. Dotted lines indicate start positions. For illustrations of machine or cable exercises, I've noted alternatives that can be done at home with dumbbells or light ankle weights.

(Any resemblance in the illustrations to a younger version of anyone real or imaginary, especially me, is purely coincidental.)

CHEST

dumbbell bench press

This exercise is great for firming and strengthening the chest, shoulders, and triceps.

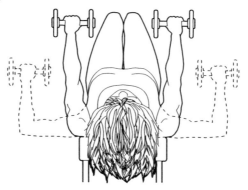

dumbbell flyes

Think chest shaper. Think cleavage.

When you do flyes, imagine that you're hugging a barrel. Not an exciting image, but it'll help your form.

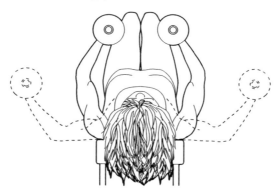

Most gyms will have a bench press machine as well as cables that can be used for flyes. Another common chest machine, often referred to as a "pec dec," is a more sophisticated version of the mail order contraptions of years ago that promised, "the bust of your dreams in six weeks or less or your money cheerfully refunded." (I'm still waiting for my check.) Good old pushups, "sissy" or regular variety, are a very effective way to work your chest without using any equipment at all.

BACK

wide grip front pulldowns
Although you may see people doing pulldowns behind the neck, the front version will help you avoid neck and shoulder strain.

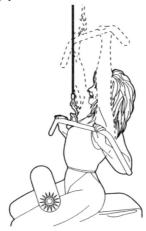

seated rows
Squeeze your shoulder blades together when you do these. Watch your form. Don't use momentum to pull the weight back.

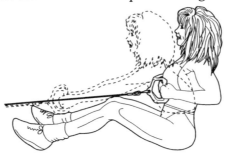

To simulate pulldowns at home, sit in a straight-back chair, hold dumbbells overhead with a slight bend in your elbows and lower slowly to shoulder level, the same position as if you were using a bar. Rows can be done with dumbbells as you lie or kneel on a bench.

SHOULDERS

overhead presses

Presses will strengthen shoulders, a weak area for many women unless they work in jobs which require hard hats.

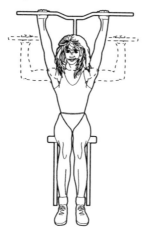

dumbbell side raises

Wonderful for shaping your shoulders, side raises may eventually eliminate the need for shoulder pads.

Overhead presses can also be done with dumbbells. Sit in a straight-back chair, hold dumbbells parallel to floor at shoulder level, elbows close to your body. Press the weights overhead. Lower slowly and repeat.

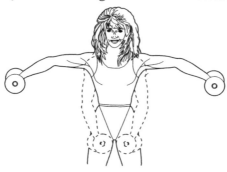

ARMS

bicep curls

Squeeze your bicep when you raise the weight and you'll really feel this exercise.

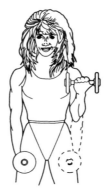

tricep kickbacks

Kickbacks will prevent saggy elephant arms.

Most gyms will have tricep pushdown and bicep curl machines. Additionally, there are different grips that you can attach to cables in order to get some variety in working these muscle groups.

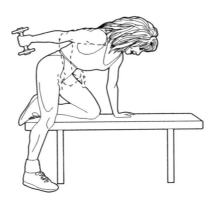

LEGS

leg extensions

Don't lock your knees when you extend. When you lower the weight, don't go beyond a 90° angle with your knees.

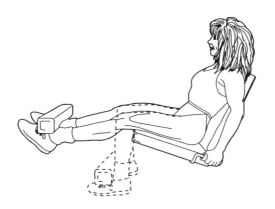

leg curls

Be careful not to arch your back as you raise your legs.

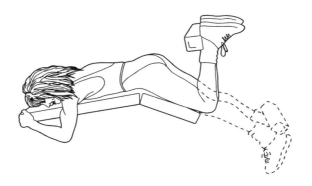

standing cable side raises

These work the outer thigh. Keep the stationary leg slightly bent.

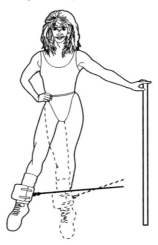

standing cable front cross kicks

These work the inner thigh. Do them right after the side raises. Remember, keep the stationary leg bent.

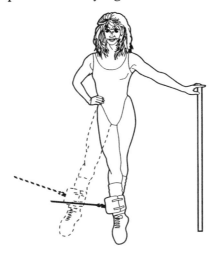

Leg extensions and leg curls can be done at home by using light ankle weights and simulating the movement of the machines. Sit in a straight-back chair for extensions. Lie prone on the floor or on a bench for curls. In the gym, look for seated leg curl machines, alternate-leg standing curl machines, and calf machines.

Side raises and cross kicks can also be done at home with light ankle weights. For outer thigh raises, lie fully extended on your left side. Raise your right leg toward the ceiling, foot flexed forward. Switch legs. For the inner thigh, assume the same position, but bend your right leg and put your right foot flat on floor in front of the left knee. Raise your left leg toward the ceiling. Switch legs.

alternate leg step up to low bench or step

Alternate leg step ups can be done on the same type of step used in aerobic step classes, on a low bench, or even on the first step of a flight of stairs. Simply step up with your right leg, then your left. Step down with your right leg, then your left. Continue in the same pattern.

standing calf raises

Holding lightly to a chair for support, go up on tiptoe. Try it one leg at a time, holding a light dumbbell in the opposite hand in order to add resistance.

If you have access to a pool, it's a good place to do leg exercises because of the water resistance.

ABDOMINALS

crunches

Be sure to keep your back flat on the floor, lifting only your shoulders. Pretend that you're holding a tennis ball between your chin and chest. To reduce back strain and isolate the abdominals, put your feet flat on the floor as in the illustration or cross them in the air.

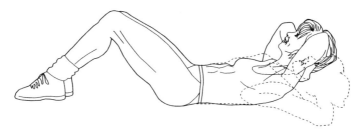

twisting crunches

To do twisting crunches, put your right foot on your left knee, keeping your left foot flat on the floor. As you lift, bring your left shoulder toward your right knee. Alternate sides.

CONSISTENCY AND CONCENTRATION

Aside from consistency, one of the biggest keys to successful weight training is concentration. In order to get the maximum benefit from the movements and not maim yourself with a dumbbell, you have to focus on your form and technique, your breathing, and the number of repetitions that you're doing.

This may seem self-evident, but you'd be surprised at how many women think that they're strength training simply because they're wearing leotards and sitting on weight resistance machines. I was intrigued by a woman who was reading a book while using an inner-outer thigh machine, a contraption that looks like something out of a gynecologist's office. From the expression on her face and the amount of time she was spending, she was either having way too much fun for the machine to be doing any good, or else she was reading something very racy. I almost broke my neck trying to get a peek at the title before I realized that she'd covered the book with a brown paper wrapper.

If you're reading while you think you're weight lifting, wake up and smell the sweat. You can't possibly do both at the same time. I must admit, however, that even though I wasn't too impressed by the way the woman on the thigh machine was training, I did take a little tip from her. I started covering my books with brown paper wrappers and labeling them with titles from Dickens and Shakespeare because I was getting sick and tired of people making smart remarks about the trashy novels that I was reading while I was on the exercise bike.

ADVANTAGES OF WEIGHT TRAINING

It's surprising how many women are unaware of the benefits of weight training. I remember one young woman at a spa who was staring at me and suddenly blurted out, "I can't believe that at your age they're not drooping." Assuming that she was talking about my breasts and not liking the age crack, I accidentally dropped a weight on her finger. Slightly appeased when I realized that she was referring to my arms, I patiently explained that it was a matter of working the biceps and triceps. After getting an ice pack for her hand, she told me how relieved she was to hear that. She'd always thought that saggy arms were hereditary. I wasn't sure what she meant until a few minutes later when her mother and grandmother walked in. Her mother had a pair of arms that had seen better days, and her grandmother's looked as if a few brisk flaps, a heavy wind, and she'd be airborne.

Not only will weight lifting keep your body parts from sagging, but larger muscles will help to fill out your skin. Typically, the only things that fill out mature skin are fluid retention and fat. However, neither of these is very aesthetic, nor can you rely on them to fill out the right spots.

Stronger muscles perform another important function. They help to keep your body parts where they were meant to be in the first place. This is not to say that weight lifting will overcome the effects of gravity, but short of plastic surgery or spending hours every day hanging upside down like a bat, it's your best bet. (Have you ever taken a close look at a bat?)

Aside from making your body more attractive, enhanced muscularity will increase your confidence because you'll be able to perform daily tasks with less effort. You'll be able to get your own luggage off airport carousels, carry your own grocery bags, change the heavy bottles on water coolers, and crush diet soda cans on your forehead.

SPECIAL BENEFITS OVER FORTY

Don't listen to people who tell you that after forty it's hopeless to try and tone your body. It may not be as simple as it was at twenty, but you've got desperation working for you. Desperation makes you more disciplined and determined than the youngsters prancing around the gym because they take what they've got for granted and you can't. You've got the dubious edge of knowing that "what youth giveth, age taketh away," and the less effort you make, the faster it goes. You also know that the better your body looks, the less people will notice your gray hair and wrinkles.

Strength training is also thought to be one of the key ways to combat **osteoporosis,** a progressive disease that causes bone tissue to deteriorate until the bones are so weak and brittle that they break under the slightest stress. In other words, you should lift weights in the hope that it'll prevent your bones from crumbling under you. Is it any wonder that we go through mid-life crisis for twenty-seven years?

I used to tease my grandmother, calling her the "incredible shrinking woman," because after a certain age she seemed to get smaller and smaller. Weight lifting can stop or slow down this degenerative process by helping you to maintain skeletal mass and upright posture. This has special significance for me since I'm not quite as tall as I tell people that I am. Getting even shorter would make me have to work that much harder at lying. I've also heard that as you get older your nose starts to droop, so theoretically, you could end up with your nostrils scraping the ground.

A study has shown that by age seventy-five, two-thirds of American women can't lift an object of more than ten pounds. This rules out many daily tasks and takes away a measure of independence. However, researchers working with residents of a center for the aged in Boston found that after eight weeks of a lower body strength training routine, most of the subjects, ranging in age from eighty-seven to ninety-six, many with arthritis, had progressed from leg-lifting an average of seventeen pounds to lifting an average of forty-two pounds. To me this screams out, "Take a look. I may be old, but I'm not dead yet!" And isn't that what it's all about?

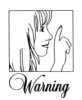

Warning

Lifting heavy weights can cause a sudden increase in blood pressure. If you have a history of heart disease or high blood pressure, get medical clearance before you begin.

HANDY LIST OF WEIGHT LIFTING WISDOM

1. Begin your weight training session with a ten minute cardiovascular warm-up followed by some light stretching. Finish your workout with some more intense stretching. Trust me on the warm-up and stretching. It's easy to cheat and leave these two steps out, but you'll pay for it.

2. While we're on the subject of stretching, contrary to the myth that weight lifting will turn you into a muscle-bound robot, performing exercises through a full range of motion will increase your flexibility. If you haven't heard the myth, do it anyway.

3. In a session, work your large muscle groups first (i.e. chest, back, or shoulders before biceps or triceps). Abdominals can be worked at the beginning or at the end of your workout.

4. No matter what kind of shape you're in or how anxious you are to improve, start slowly! Begin training with lighter weights and fewer sets, and increase gradually.

5. Before you start lifting, get some guidance in proper technique and in setting up your program.

6. Perform the exercises slowly and carefully, inhaling before you lift and exhaling on the exertion. Don't hold your breath or you'll raise your blood pressure and turn an unflattering shade of red.

7. Try to work each muscle group at least once or twice a week, but never work the same group two days in a row. Muscles need time to rest and recuperate. The only exceptions are the calves and the abdominals, which can each be worked more frequently.

9. You can relieve boredom and keep the muscles stimulated by varying your routine with free weights (dumbbells and barbells), machines, and body weight (i.e. push ups).

10. A modest amount of weight training three times a week can drastically improve your appearance. Studies have shown that over a period of time, by doing two lower body exercises and six upper body exercises, women have lost an average of three pounds of fat and gained three pounds of muscle. Though their weight didn't change (muscle tissue is denser than fat), their body composition was significantly altered. Many of them lost an inch around the waist and dropped fat off of their thighs.

Chapter 8

Flexibility Over Forty: Fact or Fiction?

FLEXIBILITY

I used to get very defensive when anyone would suggest that I should be more flexible. I thought it was their way of informing me that I needed an attitude adjustment. How was I supposed to know they were referring to stretching? But believe me, an attitude adjustment is nothing compared to making your body more flexible. Unless you're one of those unusually supple women who could probably get work as a circus contortionist (my husband wanted to know if I was so into exercise, why I couldn't be more like those women), it's going to take time and perseverance to get your body parts to move like they should and probably once did.

A BRIEF HISTORY OF STRETCHING

Stretching is not a new concept. We can look as far back as the fifteenth century to find the prototype for the stretching machines that are constantly being peddled on late night television. Known as the "rack," it was used to torture people by stretching them between rollers set into a frame. Granted, it was more extreme than most modern versions, but it taught us a cardinal rule of exercise—never stretch to the point of pain.

Unlike the rack, the purpose of modern stretching is to improve your range of motion, not to tear your joints out of their sockets. In order to move your joints freely and painlessly through this wider range, you have to stretch the muscles around them regularly. This should always be done with gentle and relaxing movements.

STRETCHING—THE CONDOM OF EXERCISE

Stretching is often the most overlooked part of a fitness program because it's so easy to skip it. When you're all warmed up and ready to run, bike, or swim, who wants to take the time to stop and stretch? It would be as if you were about to have sex and your partner said, "Let's take a few minutes to limber up first." It's not a bad idea, it just calls for self-discipline. You can regard stretching as the condom of exercise. It takes a little extra effort, but it protects your body from unnecessary harm.

THE BODY IS A COMPLICATED MACHINE

I heard a yoga teacher use an analogy that vividly emphasized the importance of stretching. She said, "If you think of the body as a machine with moveable parts, when the parts stop moving, the machine breaks down." She told me this as I was trying to convince her that my machine had rusted and couldn't possibly accomplish what she expected it to. What I actually said was, "You want me to put my foot where... while my arms are wrapped around my what?" I suggested that it would be much easier just to throw on a little WD-40 or to send my body to the shop for a lube job. Not only wouldn't she buy it, but then she turned her torso around at such an extreme angle, it looked as if her head was on backward. It was like watching *The Exorcist.*

NATURAL LIMITS

Not everyone has the same degree of natural flexibility, so you have to work to improve within your limits. You may be very envious of the woman who can turn inside out, but we can't all be Gumby (besides, Gumby is green and funny looking). You also have to keep in mind that unless you've stretched consistently over the years, you've probably lost quite a bit of the flexibility that you used to have. You can find it again, but it's going to be a gradual process that takes some work.

❧❧❧

PERSONAL ANECDOTE: "SPLITS ARE FOR KIDS"

Ignoring that last bit of advice, and not having done a backbend in more years than I care to admit (although I was very proficient at them as a double-jointed child), I decided to try one. I will only say that my husband scraped me up off the floor and deposited me in my car, figuring that in case I could never move again, at least I'd be able to drive carpool.

I had a similar but more positive experience with doing splits. When one of my friends wagered that I'd never be able to do a split (another of my childhood feats), I smugly informed her that I'd be glad to take her money. Hedging her bet, she added the stipulation that it had to be in this lifetime. Not one to give up easily and having learned a valuable lesson from my backbend fiasco, I began practicing every day and acquired some other important lessons. First, if you don't take a few minutes to warm up before stretching, it's painful, dangerous, and nearly impossible. Second, mature, sensible women should not be doing splits. And third, I should have kept my big mouth shut. Nevertheless, I'm happy to report that after six months I got those splits back again and was able to get up off the floor and walk away.

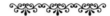

THE BASIC PRINCIPLES OF STRETCHING

The following are points to remember in order to stretch safely and effectively, and to keep your body from getting stuck in positions that make it impossible for you to leave the house.

1. Warm up before you limber up. Before you even think about stretching, warm up by doing something aerobic for five to ten minutes.
2. Find a comfortable spot on the floor and pretend that you like what you're doing.
3. Inhale and move slowly and gently into each stretch. Exhale as you feel the muscles extend.
4. Hold each stretch for fifteen to twenty seconds without bouncing.
5. Rest briefly (try not to fall asleep) and repeat the cycle three to five times.
6. Stretch before, during, and after your workouts. The initial stretching is intended to work your muscles through their range of motion. The final stretching is to increase flexibility so it should be more intense.
7. Stretch daily.
8. If you've never done a split in your life, now is not the time to start unless someone offers you a large sum of money.
9. Stretch within your natural limits, not the limits of some show-off who may be working next to you.

10. Consistent stretching, no matter how inconvenient, will protect you from unnecessary injury.
11. Never stretch to the point of pain.

Pain is subjective. One woman's labor may be another's scrape on the knee, so be sensible. When stretching, a slight pulling is okay; a sharp burning sensation isn't. If you find yourself moaning or screaming out in pain, immediately stop what you're doing.

BASIC STRETCHES
The following are some suggested stretches to help you relax from head to toe.

Standing Stretches
Whenever you do standing stretches, keep your feet shoulder width apart and your knees slightly bent.

The first three stretches are effective alternatives to half neck circles.

Head side to side. Look right then left, remembering to hold each position for fifteen to twenty seconds.

Ear to shoulder. Tilt your right ear toward your right shoulder, without lifting your shoulder. Hold, then tilt to the other side.

Chin to chest. Lower your chin to your chest and hold. Don't reverse this stretch because stretching your head back will put too much strain on the cervical vertebrae in your neck.

Shrug. This is just what it sounds like and is also the appropriate response to anyone who interrupts to ask why you're doing this.

Alternate arm overhead reach. Extend arms overhead, reach right then left as if trying to grab the last pair of shoes off the top shelf of the sale rack.

Arm across chest stretch. This is a pleasant stretch because you hug yourself at the same time that you're relaxing your shoulders and upper back. Use your hand to hold your arm, not to push on your elbow. Alternate sides.

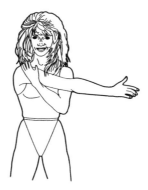

Chest stretch against the wall. This is a simple yet effective stretch for your chest, shoulders, and arms. Gently turn your torso further away from the wall to increase the effect. Alternate sides.

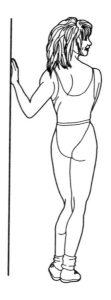

Calf stretch against the wall. Face the wall. Standing about three feet back, lean into the wall with both hands at shoulder level. Bring your right leg forward with knee bent. Extend your left leg straight back and press your heel into the floor until you feel a stretch in the calf. Switch legs.

Seated Stretches

Butterfly. This is very effective for your inner thighs and hips. To increase flexibility, gently press down on your knees.

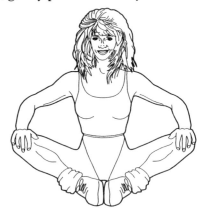

Modified hurdler. Equally as effective as the traditional hurdler stretch, this is much easier on your knees.

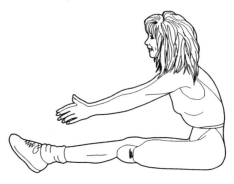

Forward hamstring. This is a safe replacement for standing toe touch-es. Sit on the floor with legs extended in front of you. Keeping your knees slightly bent and your back flat, reach toward your toes.

Straddle. Sit in the same position as for the previous stretch, but strad-dle your legs. Keeping your knees relaxed and your back flat, turn your torso to the right and reach for your toes. Reverse to the left. If you're more limber, you can also reach for the floor in front of you.

Back twist. This stretch helps your hips and lower back. You can increase the effect by slowly turning your torso a little bit further. Alter-nate sides.

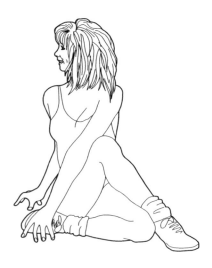

Reclining Stretches

Knee to chest. Lying on your back, bring your right knee to your chest. Put your hands under your right thigh and pull gently. Switch legs. You can also do this with both legs at the same time.

Leg cross-over. This stretch relaxes your back as well as your glutes. Remember to turn your head in the opposite direction from the crossed over leg.

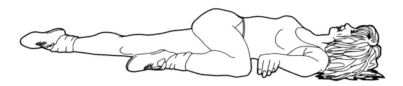

Whole body stretch. This is a perfect finishing stretch. Lie flat on the floor with legs straight and arms overhead. Tense your body, pushing your hands in one direction and your feet in the other. Now you can relax and fall asleep.

Some Stretches Can Be Hazardous to Your Health

Just as splits or backbends may not be for you, there are other common stretches that you should avoid.

Standing toe touch. Do we even need to discuss how this feels on your back and knees? Take a seat and do it with your legs slightly bent.

Hurdler stretch. Runners often use this stretch (one leg straight in front, the other bent back) to loosen up their legs, but it's tough on knees. Do the modified version instead.

Full neck circles. Full circles cause hypertension of the neck and put too much stress on the vertebral column. Besides, my neck sounds like a bowl of Rice Krispies when I do them, and that gives me the creeps. Replace them with half neck rolls, side to side head turns, ear to shoulder, and chin to chest movements.

Backbend. As you recall, this movement nearly put me out of commission. Try the knee to chest stretch instead, or get on your hands and knees, curl your back like a cat, then relax it. Be very careful not to arch.

Plough. This is a yoga stretch in which you lie on your back and try to put your legs over your head. Aside from the fact that this can cause neck and back problems, it looks extremely undignified.

Cobra. This is a yoga posture in which you hyperextend your back from a prone position. I refuse to have anything to do with snakes, but if you feel the need to do the cobra, play it safe by keeping your elbows and abdomen on the floor.

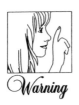

Avoid any stretch where you feel sensation, particularly unpleasant sensation, in the joint rather than the muscle.

Warning

Chapter 9

You Are
What You Eat—
Except When
You Have PMS

THE NUTRITION OBSESSION

Although eating right is a relatively simple concept—putting the right amount of the right fuel into your body—it's become a national preoccupation. We obsess about what to eat, what not to eat, how much, and how little. We further complicate it by using food as an emotional Band-Aid, drowning our sorrows in quarts of ice cream and burying stress under piles of potato chips.

Before going any further, let's take a few moments to put the whole subject in perspective. First, study the word **nutrition**. Notice anything unusual? The first three letters are **n-u-t**, and that's exactly what you're going to be if you let your diet run your life. Now take a closer look at the word diet. Oddly enough, the first three letters are **d-i-e**, precisely what you're going to feel like doing if you try to follow a regimen that's too extreme and spend half your waking hours thinking about all of the food that you shouldn't be eating.

While we're on the subject of words, let me call your attention to the first three letters of **bean**, one of the main staples of a vegetarian diet. **B-e-a** may not mean much to you, but I have a great aunt named Bea who is one of the biggest fruit loops in my family, and I don't have a family that's known for being normal. I have no problem with vegetarians if they practice sensibly and leave me alone, but this coincidence with Bea is a bit unnerving.

EATING JUNK FOOD SHOWS

Now that we have that out of the way, lets get down to the nitty gritty. There's no denying that proper nutrition is vital to your health and crucial to your appearance. You can exercise until you're ready to drop, but if you're eating junk, it's going to show, no matter if you're overweight or thin and flabby. Get naked, stand in front of a mirror (with the doors to the room double-bolted, of course), and you'll see exactly where the gravy, cookies, and deep-fried foods went. You'll be able to find the lumpy areas that sucked in fat like a vacuum cleaner. You can pay a doctor to do liposuction and suck it all back out again, but that's expensive and fairly disgusting. Have you ever seen what human fat looks like? It's so repulsive that keeping a jar of it on the kitchen counter would cut down on compulsive snacking.

THE CELLULITE DEMON

As if being over forty doesn't already carry enough baggage, it's also the time when the cellulite demon attacks with a vengeance. Though he can strike at any age, he seems to have a distinct preference for older women. He makes sure that you pay for eating too much or for eating the wrong foods. (This isn't the same demon who gives you heartburn and indigestion, but they often work as a team.) Coincidentally, the cellulite demon seems to be more active in the summer, just when you'd hoped to be able to wear a bathing suit in public without getting arrested for indecent exposure.

If you don't buy the demon theory, here's another explanation for cellulite. As you get older you naturally carry more fat. A pound of fat takes up twenty percent more room than a pound of muscle. At the same time, your skin and other connective tissue lose some of their elasticity, so you often end up with ugly bulges and ripples. Cellulite is not "special" fat as some people would lead you to believe, unless you consider fatty deposits under the skin that give you unattractive dimpling to be special.

DESPERATION CAN BE DANGEROUS

The desperate desire to find the answer to staying thin and cellulite low (free would be nice, but let's be realistic) can inspire normally sensible women to do very odd things and to follow pointless eating regimens. If you want a prime example, consider the number of women in this country with anorexia and bulimia. Even though these eating disorders are really dangerous illnesses, they've become very common.

There are millions of other women who won't go to that extreme, but who'd be more than willing to try something slightly less drastic if there was even a remote chance that it might be effective. If someone over forty with a "to-die-for" body revealed that her secret was to eat while standing on one foot and wearing dirty sweat socks, there are legions of women who'd give it a try. They'd figure it couldn't hurt, it might help, and it would certainly cut down on laundry.

"THE EXPERTS"

Using this element of desperation to their advantage are the self-proclaimed experts who have no idea what they're talking about. Sometimes it seems that anyone who's ever consumed a meal containing more than one of the main food groups thinks that she's an authority on nutrition. (For the edification of one of my daughters—she knows which one she is—the main food groups are not dessert, fried foods, pretzels, and beer.)

Even authentic experts can load you up with so much confusing and conflicting information that you won't know what to do. Some will tell you that you have to combine protein and carbohydrates in one meal. Others will insist that you keep them totally separate or even eat them in a particular order. I'd like to know how you're supposed to know which theory to believe and how to keep all the data straight.

As if combining the right foods isn't confusing enough, there are other authorities who'll tell you when you should be eating what. As far as I can figure, they're a bunch of morning people because they get very specific about breakfast, advising you to measure each mouthful and count every calorie. I agree that breakfast is an important meal since the body has gone all night without nourishment or fuel, but first thing in the a.m., I'm lucky if my shoes are on the right feet and I'm not wearing my husband's underwear.

WARNING: DIETS ARE HAZARDOUS TO YOUR HEALTH

Along the same lines, let's talk about fad diets and crash diets. They're depressing, punishing, and counter-productive. They're the invention of self-promoters who want to sell you diet food, a diet program, their latest diet book, or all three. They lure you in with outrageous promises and before and after photos out of your dreams. I'm sorry, but a diet won't transform you from a short, dumpy brunette to a statuesque blonde with an eighteen inch waist.

By the time you've read the books, tried the diets, lost the weight and gained it back again, the perpetrators have skipped town with the royalties. They're on cruises to the Bahamas, wolfing down everything in sight. These opportunists are no strangers to room service and the buffet table, which is why they had to come up with diets in the first place.

Diet Centers

The more responsible diet centers may work for you if you can't do it on your own or if you enjoy having to weigh in regularly, but they're not for everyone. My friend went to a weight loss center and bought her quota for the week. Unfortunately, she polished off the week's supply in an afternoon. When she went back for a refill and tried to convince the diet police that her dog had attacked the bag, they said they were sure her dog would never stoop so low. Then they forced her to get on the scale while they all stood around shaking their heads and making faces. I would rather tape my mouth shut for a week than endure that humiliation.

⁂

True Confession (Okay, it's a Personal Anecdote.)

In clear conscience, I must admit that I've been on diets in the past, usually in preparation for bodybuilding competition. Knowing almost nothing about nutrition or dieting when I started out, I naively turned to the muscle-bound hulks in the gym for advice. Big mistake. One insisted that I eat only chicken, codfish, and potatoes. Another expert said that I should stick to tuna, melon, and cottage cheese. I told him to go stick to a wall.

Utterly confused and frustrated, but also desperate, I tried each of their suggestions and never wanted to eat again. I'd walk into the supermarket and hear the candy bars calling my name. I'd have dreams about dinners in fine restaurants and nightmares about chickens trying to peck my eyes out. I was afraid to go to the beach because I was sure I'd cry if I saw one more fish, or the fish would cry if they saw me. The moment I began a diet I was miserable and the second that I finished competing, I'd head straight for the greasiest food that I could slide my teeth into.

Finally I asked myself, "What's wrong with this picture? I'm supposed to be a healthy athlete (I love saying that), but instead I'm alternating between dumb diets and junk food orgies." I realized that what

97

was missing, aside from a few brain cells that had been wiped out by the diets and one too many days in the gym, was balance.

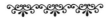

THE BALANCED APPROACH TO EATING

Going to extremes with eating simply doesn't work. It's hard on your body and on your psyche. You're not going to get the job done by starving yourself (your body will lower its metabolic rate as if there was real famine, making it more difficult to burn fat), eating very limited types of food, or jumping on and off the scale every three hours to see if you've lost an ounce.

If you're trying to lose weight, taking off a pound or two a week is the reasonable thing to do. If you lose too quickly by going too low on your calorie intake, you'll probably gain it back again, with interest. In addition, you'll lose lean weight, put back fatty weight, and again slow down your metabolism. After several diets, even though you may weigh what you did at senior prom, your percentage of body fat will be higher.

A moderate approach may not be thrilling, but neither is brushing your teeth, and most of us do that on a regular basis. Just like exercising, eating right has to become a habit, not something that you do to excess and only when the mood strikes.

THE OFFICIAL WORD—THE PYRAMID

If you're looking for a place to start, you can turn to the Food Group Pyramid. Approved by the USDA and the National Center for Nutrition and Dietetics, the pyramid replaces the once familiar Basic Food Group Wheel in setting the standard for a balanced daily diet. Although you can find the pyramid on many common food packages, it's usually too small for anyone over forty to see. Refer to the illustration in this chapter instead.

The broad base of the pyramid puts the emphasis on eating bread, rice, cereal, and pasta, followed by fruits and vegetables—foods which supply vitamins, minerals, complex carbohydrates, and dietary fiber. Next in importance come the meat, fish, dry beans, eggs, and nuts group, significant sources of the protein which is necessary to build muscle and maintain tissue, and the milk, yogurt, and cheese group. Wouldn't you know it? Fats, oils, and sweets are only allotted a small space at the tip of the pyramid.

Aside from spelling out the ideal proportion for each food group, the pyramid also indicates a preferred number of daily servings. You'll notice that fats, oils, and sweets aren't even dignified by a recommended number. You'd be consuming about 1600 calories a day with the lowest number of portions and about 2800 with the highest. Incidentally, 1200 calories per day is the minimum I'd advise for healthy, long-lasting weight loss.

Although trying to eat all of the recommended servings may seem a bit overwhelming, I'm including the pyramid for a few reasons:

- It's an excellent point of reference if you have no idea what type of food you should be eating.
- It's a clear way to see the proportions and the amounts of the various foods that you should be eating.
- It offers practical suggestions for servings from each group.
- Pyramids have good karma.

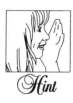

Hint

For easy measuring, your palm will hold approximately three ounces of meat. If you're trying to impress people with your table manners and don't want to pick up food in your hands, you can also assume that a three ounce serving of meat is about the size of a deck of cards.

Substitute low or non-fat dairy products in the milk, yogurt, cheese group, and substitute egg whites for whole eggs. By eliminating the yolks, you'll be getting protein without all of the fat.

Under bread, cereal etc., select whole-grain varieties. Just because bread is brown doesn't necessarily mean that it's whole grain, so check the ingredients.

𝓕ood 𝓟yramid

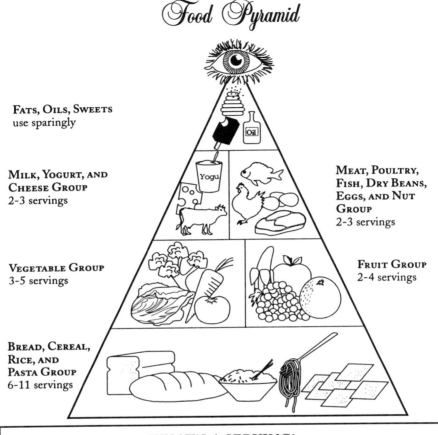

Fats, Oils, Sweets
use sparingly

Milk, Yogurt, and Cheese Group
2-3 servings

Meat, Poultry, Fish, Dry Beans, Eggs, and Nut Group
2-3 servings

Vegetable Group
3-5 servings

Fruit Group
2-4 servings

Bread, Cereal, Rice, and Pasta Group
6-11 servings

WHAT'S A SERVING?

Bread, Cereal, Rice, and Pasta
1 slice bread, dinner roll, or
  ½ hamburger bun
1 ounce ready-to-eat cereal
½ cup cooked rice, cereal, or pasta

Vegetables
1 cup raw leafy vegetables
½ cup raw or cooked chopped vegetables
¾ cup vegetable juice

Milk, Yogurt, Cheese
1 cup milk or yogurt
1½ ounces natural cheese
2 ounces processed cheese

Fruit
1 medium apple, orange, or banana
½ cup cooked or canned fruit
¾ cup fruit juice

Meat, Poultry, Fish, Dry Beans, Eggs, and Nuts
2–3 ounces cooked lean meat, poultry,
  or fish
1–1½ cups cooked dry beans
1 egg or 1 tablespoon peanut butter
  counts as the equivalent of 1 ounce
  of meat (use sparingly because of
  cholesterol and fat)

Source: U.S. Department of Agriculture, U.S. Department of Health and Human Services

EASY EATING RULES

My approach to eating is quite basic. Instead of weighing and measuring each bite that I put into my mouth, which would be too much work and force me to spend an inordinate amount of time thinking about food, I just follow a few simple rules (always bearing in mind that rules are made to be broken in case someone waves a piece of chocolate cake in front of my face). These rules aren't unusual or unique, but they're practical, easy to remember, and effective.

RULE #1—WATCH YOUR FAT INTAKE.

Above all, watch your fats! There are no two ways about it, to stay fit and healthy, you have to keep your intake of fats, especially saturated fats such as lard, butter, tropical oils (palm kernel and coconut), and hydrogenated oils, low. (Saturated fats are usually solid at room temperature.) Since many experts suggest that fat should make up only ten to fifteen percent of your diet, staying under twenty percent is a reasonable goal for most women.

To be more specific, find twenty percent of your daily caloric intake and divide this by nine (the number of calories in a gram of fat as opposed to four calories in a gram of protein or carbohydrates). This will give you your maximum daily allowance of grams of fat. For example:

$$1{,}800 \text{ calories} \times .20 = 360 \text{ calories}$$
$$360 \text{ calories} \div 9 = 40 \text{ grams of fat}$$

Once you've determined your maximum number of grams, pay attention to what you're eating so that you stay within the limit. This is much easier than it used to be because everything is labeled. All you have to do is read packages, closely noting serving size, percentage of various nutrients, as well as the ingredients, which are listed in decreasing order of content. You can also purchase an inexpensive fat counter book which lists fat content of most common foods.

Warning

Beware of products that use tiny print. They're hiding something from you.

Be on your guard with so called non-fat products. They may contain traces of fat which can add up if you consume a huge portion. By the same token, always make careful note of portion size. What the manufacturer calls a full serving may not even be enough to satisfy a pet hamster. The recommended serving of some non-fat cakes is so thin that you can see through the slice.

Also bear in mind that non-fat foods may be loaded with sugar, salt, chemicals, or other empty calories, all of which you should keep to a minimum. Eating a fat-free cookie is preferable to eating one that's loaded with saturated fat, but the words "fat-free" are not synonymous with "consume the whole box."

RULE #2—BALANCE YOUR DIET.

As suggested in the pyramid, keep your diet balanced, putting the emphasis on carbohydrates such as fruits, vegetables, and whole grains. If you do a lot of weight lifting, consume a little extra protein to help rebuild muscle. This doesn't imply that you should polish off a side of beef after every workout, but a helping of chicken or fish wouldn't hurt.

Also balance your eating with your level of exercise. If you're inactive for a period of time, cut back on your food intake because you won't be burning as many calories.

RULE #3—EAT SEVERAL MINI-MEALS A DAY.

Recently, someone at the gym referred to me as a "grazer." Assuming that he was comparing me to a cow, I kicked him with my hoof and then asked him what he meant by that. When he explained that he was referring to my habit of eating small amounts of food all day long, about five or six mini-meals as opposed to three full meals, I agreed that it was bovine behavior but still wasn't thrilled with the analogy.

Despite the implications, I believe that grazing is a much easier and more healthful way to eat. It keeps your blood sugar level balanced which prevents you from getting so ravenous that you want to consume the entire contents of your house. You burn food more efficiently and don't feel depressed or hostile because of food deprivation. However, if you miss those emotions, I'm sure you can find other ways to conjure them up. For example, try watching a teenage girl wolf down a burger and fries without one shred of guilt and without gaining an ounce.

Using the pyramid is an easy way to plan five small meals. Select the servings that you want and then spread them out over the course of the day, making sure to include breakfast. I mention this because like so many women I used to skip breakfast, figuring that the longer I could go without eating, the better off I'd be. Wrong! Skipping breakfast causes you to consume more food later on in the day and deprives your body of nourishment at an essential time.

Rule #4—Leave the table before you're full.

If you're so stuffed after a meal that Macy's wants to put you up in the air for their Thanksgiving parade, you don't need a calorie count to let you know that you've eaten too much. I'm convinced that most women know when they're overeating. They're just enjoying themselves too much to stop or have nothing better to do. If you fall into the second category, get a hobby.

Rule #5—Drink six to eight glasses of water a day.

Water is vital for your health. It helps metabolize stored fat, maintain proper muscle tone, and flush your system. Keep in mind, however, that your system isn't the only thing that'll be flushing. Be sure that you're never too far from a bathroom.

Rule #6—PMS cancels all of the other rules.

If you're experiencing PMS or some other temporary problem, such as an extended visit from your mother-in-law, that's wreaking havoc with your best intentions, you can break the rules without guilt. A slight lapse every now and then is not the end of the world.

EATING TIPS THAT REALLY WORK

After hearing my rules, women often wink knowingly and ask, "Don't you have any real eating secrets to share?" as if to imply that I've made a pact with the devil to stay in shape (not that I wouldn't if I thought it would help). Actually I do have several other tips that may be of more value to you than anything else in this entire chapter.

TIP #1. BE PREPARED—DON'T LEAVE HOME WITHOUT FOOD.

The surest way to find yourself in line at a fast food restaurant is to be out and about when hunger strikes. You'll be tempted to go for the quickest, easiest thing you can grab, no matter how much of a nutritional disaster it may be. Whether you're going to be taking care of business, shopping, working out, or robbing convenience stores, consider bringing a baked potato, fresh fruits or vegetables, zip-top cans of tuna packed in water, chicken breasts, rice cakes or whole grain rolls, and of course, a large bottle of water. On long days, keep a small cooler of food in the car.

TIP #2. IF YOU DON'T WANT TO EAT IT, GET IT AWAY FROM YOU.

Say you're out to dinner and an incredible dessert is being served. You're torn between replying "no thank you," or tackling the waiter and grabbing six off the tray. My advice is to wait until you're served, have a few bites so that you don't feel deprived, then get that sucker as far away from you as possible. Give it to someone else at the table, slide it under your chair or drop kick it across the room. Put it where you can't reach it!

TIP #3. ALONG THE SAME LINES, IF THERE'S SOMETHING THAT YOU KNOW YOU SHOULDN'T BE EATING, DON'T KEEP IT IN THE HOUSE.

Eating right is tough enough without having temptation sitting in your kitchen. Don't kid yourself into thinking that you can buy a big bag of chocolate kisses, store it in the freezer, and allow yourself only one or two a day. Unless you've got the will power of a thin pastry chef, you're setting yourself up for a high fat fall.

TIP #4. KEEP ALTERNATIVE SNACKS ON HAND.

It's easier to stop eating the wrong foods if the right ones are available. The following suggestions are for snacks that, if not perfect, are at least preferable:

- fresh fruits and vegetables—frozen grapes and bananas may satisfy a sweet tooth
- pretzels instead of chips
- toasted bagels with fruit spread, instead of muffins
- non-fat frozen yogurt or frozen fruit bars instead of ice cream
- fruit shakes (fresh fruit, non-fat milk, and ice)
- low-fat granola cereal and granola bars
- air-popped popcorn and rice cakes (also effective as packing material)
- graham crackers instead of cookies

TIP #5. DON'T BE AFRAID TO MAKE SPECIAL REQUESTS AT RESTAURANTS.

When you're out to eat, don't hesitate to ask that your meal be prepared with little or no oil, with less salt, or with dressings and sauces on the side. What's the chef going to do—come after you with a meat cleaver or spit on your food? My husband and kids used to roll their eyes and try to hide under the table when it was my turn to order. Let me tell you, they've all gotten rather picky themselves.

TIP #6. SHARE FOOD.

Another helpful idea at restaurants is to share food, preferably with someone in your party. Split an entree in two or get one dessert and several forks for the entire table. Portions are frequently too large. (You're served the same meal as a pro linebacker.) As for dessert, a taste is often better than none at all.

TIP #7. PRACTICE DAMAGE CONTROL AT FAST FOOD RESTAURANTS.

If some irresistible force drives you to a fast food restaurant, try the following substitutions:

- grilled chicken instead of fried chicken or a greasy burger
- plain baked potato instead of fries or a baked potato that's fully loaded; season with low or non-fat dressing
- salad with dressing on the side as opposed to one that's pre-mixed
- ketchup and mustard as condiments rather than mayonnaise or other fatty spreads
- small (even kiddie) servings instead of jumbo, mansize, el grande, or whatever else they're called

TIP #8. PUT YOUR CRAVINGS ON HOLD.

If you have a yen for a particular food that's going to put inches on your hips, cause instant acne, or make your hands and feet swell, attempt to distract yourself. I've heard that if you wait twenty minutes, a craving will usually disappear, but I think it depends on what you're doing during those twenty minutes. Staring into the refrigerator isn't going to work unless someone slams your head in the door. Try tweezing your eyebrows, paying bills, or searching for new gray hairs. If all of that pain doesn't make the craving vanish, figure it was meant to be.

If this happens once in awhile, don't feel guilty and beat yourself up. Giving in to an occasional craving is better than eating circles around it and still coming back to it in the end. If this happens to you several times a day, or if you start to enjoy beating yourself up, you might want to seek professional help.

TIP #9. IDENTIFY AND CHANGE YOUR NEGATIVE EATING PATTERNS.

If, like millions of other people, you finish dinner and then spend the rest of the evening making trips into the kitchen, change your routine. Watch TV in a different room (preferably one that's further from the refrigerator). Go for a walk instead of settling into your usual spot on the sofa. Do whatever it takes to break the pattern.

The same holds true if you lose your resolve at some other time of the day or in some other way. Identify your pattern and change it. If you have a tendency to overeat in the car, don't keep food in the front seat with you. (Besides, how can you apply makeup, talk on the phone, and drive if you're eating?) If your nutrition suffers from lack of planning, write out a menu for yourself. If food is your cure for depression, try getting comfort from a friend instead of from a french fry.

Tip #10. Stop eating after seven p.m.

There is no reason to load up with food right before you go to sleep unless you're planning on hibernating.

Tip #11. Revise your recipes.

When you're forced to cook (Have I given myself away?), find ways to downscale the fat, sugar, and salt in your recipes. It's surprisingly easy to substitute non-fat products for regular, egg whites for whole eggs (use one or two extra), herbs and spices for salt, and natural sweeteners for processed sugar. Just don't tell your family what you're up to or they'll swear they can taste the difference. Then again, if you're looking for a way out of the kitchen, whip up a few non-fat, non-sugar, non-salt, non-flavor meals and you'll be home free.

Tip #12. Keep a food diary.

Occasionally, write down every single morsel of food that you put in your mouth over a three or four day period. If you're honest, the embarrassment alone will stop you from pigging out. This method will also help you identify any food intolerance that you may have and will enable you to pinpoint problem areas in your diet.

Tip #13. Chew sugarless gum while you're cooking.

If you think walking and chewing gum at the same time is difficult, try simultaneously tasting out of the pot and chomping on a wad of gum.

Tip #14. Drink a few glasses of water or eat some fresh fruit before going to a party.

This will usually fill you up enough to keep you from pouncing on the hors d'oeuvres.

Tip #15. Don't eat when you're bored.

Boredom is not a sign of hunger. If you're bored, find something to do, not something to eat.

Tip #16. Break the rules every now and then.

If your diet is consistently well-balanced, low-fat, and moderate calorie, give yourself an occasional treat. You might even want to designate one day a week as your "indulgence day," a time to eat anything you'd like **within reason.**

Think of it as an incentive program for exemplary behavior. This will also prevent you from becoming an eating saint, and after all, no one is really comfortable dealing with saints on a daily basis. Like complaining in the gym, not having perfect eating habits makes you much more likable.

Chapter 10

Taming the
Stress Monster

WHAT IS STRESS?

Stress is the way your body reacts to new or unusual situations, whether welcome or unwelcome. Your heart beats faster, your body produces adrenaline (a natural stimulant), you breathe more rapidly, are more alert, and may perspire more. All of these responses can work for you (think of the competitive edge when you're fighting the crowds at storewide sales), but only in limited doses and followed by periods of relaxation.

Problems set in when your body remains in that heightened state and can't unwind—when you let everything get to you and put way too much pressure on yourself. Then stress becomes the enemy, causing a myriad of symptoms that would seem to have no logical explanation. Stress can make you overeat or undereat, undersleep or oversleep, feel sick, anxious, or sore. It can cause pimples, hives, rashes, or gas.

Uncontrolled stress is like a stubborn fungus—annoying, undesirable, and persistent. It's like a hangnail that you have to keep cutting off or pushing back in order to keep it under control. Have you ever noticed how psychologists talk about stress management rather than stress elimination, implying that since you're stuck with it, you may as well learn how to live with it?

Good News

Working out is one of the best ways to cage the stress monster. In a sense, exercise replaces psychic stress with more beneficial physical stress. Aside from providing a positive outlet for rechanneling your negative energy and causing the release of uplifting endorphins, working out can also leave you so exhausted that you won't have the strength to worry about your problems.

No matter what your mood, a few minutes into exercising you should feel about ten times better than you did when you started. After getting stuck in an express check-out lane behind people who think that having eighteen items is about the same as having ten, or listening to your daughter explain why she'll be moving back in with you so that she can give up her job at the law firm and become a street musician, there's nothing like an hour in the gym to blow off a little steam.

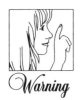

Warning

To the contrary, over-exercising, instead of eliminating stress, may put too many demands on your body and cause unnecessary strain. Working out can help you cope, but it can't provide all of the answers. It has to be approached sensibly. You should feel pleasantly fatigued when you finish a session, not ready for hospitalization.

A fitness program can also kick in a little stress of its own. You have to worry about quitting your job and abandoning your family so that you can find time for all of your activities, eating properly, avoiding injuries, affording the latest in leotards, and obsessing over your body. If overdone, it's enough to turn even the sanest woman into a neurotic mess.

STRESS BUSTERS

If you find that consistent exercise and proper nutrition are helping with your physical stress, but aren't quite doing it for your emotional and psychic strain, there are a number of other avenues to explore. Try one of the following options to soothe your soul or whatever else needs soothing.

YOGA

Yoga, which I also referred to under stretching, is an effective means to calm your mind as well as your body. You can achieve a general sense of relaxation as you release the muscle tightness which is often associated with stress.

There are many different styles of yoga, some emphasizing the mental discipline and others the physical. Again, be sure to find out what you're getting into and which you prefer. Some classes are also much more rigorous than others and may be too demanding for your level of fitness. Personally, I don't want to spend much time standing on my head and breathing through my "third eye," but if this sounds like your cup of herbal tea, then go for it. My preference is for classes that offer gentle but thorough stretching and deep breathing through the normal body parts. I enrolled in one class that was so soothing, the teacher had to keep waking me up because my snoring was disturbing everyone else.

I suggest that you find a teacher who's your age or even older. Older ones understand the struggle to retain or regain flexibility. Do you really want to be taught by some young rubber band who does pretzel impressions as a warm-up? Older teachers also feel the little aches and pains and aren't afraid to complain, which should make you feel much more secure. If you encounter one who's unusually limber for her age, view it as inspiration rather than as a threat to your well-being.

Yoga classes at health clubs are a reliable choice for the beginner. They're usually designed for the average person who wants to relieve tension and improve flexibility with slow stretching and deep breathing. The instructors will teach the basic yoga postures with a real concern for safety because health clubs pay huge insurance premiums and can't afford to have too many members put in traction.

MEDITATION

Many people have the misconception that meditation is a mystical practice left over from the hippie era and that you have to be out in "La La Land" to do it. Thanks to the technique, you'll no longer care what they think.

Meditation is a method of clearing thoughts, particularly stressful thoughts, from your mind. It provides an escape hatch from daily hassles and allows you to stop and take time out instead of overreacting to pressure.

A form of mental exercise, in some ways it's very similar to a program of physical exercise. The activity itself may seem silly (think about weight lifting—you keep picking up an object and putting it back down again as if you can't make up your mind), but it has valuable long-term, cumulative effects. Also like physical disciplines, it should be adapted to the individual and performed consistently in order to achieve the best results.

There are several different ways to learn how to meditate. You can:

- Drop out and travel to India, the Himalayas, or some other exotic locale.
- Hire your own personal guru.
- Buy a secret mantra or chant.
- Take classes at a community education center, yoga school, or health club.
- Buy a straightforward book such as *How to Meditate* by Lawrence LeShan or a guided meditation tape at a new age metaphysical book store (you know, the ones with incense, wind chimes, and other-worldly sales people).

A Taste of Meditation

Here are two basic exercises that will offer you a taste of meditation. They may sound easy, but give them a try if you want to see how truly difficult it is to make your mind relax.

1. Sit comfortably in a quiet place. (You can try the cross-legged or lotus position, but it's not necessary and for some women it's not even feasible). Focus on your breathing, inhaling and exhaling slowly. Begin counting breaths, going only up to four and then starting again with one. When your mind wanders (and it will), simply bring your attention back to your breathing. Set a timer and see if you can keep this up for a minute or two.
2. Watch something restful that captures your attention such as ocean waves, cloud formations, or trees blowing in the wind. Don't think about what you're seeing—just see it (like you do with television). If you catch yourself trying to think, force yourself back to just seeing. Try to do this for a few minutes at a time.

Performing either of these exercises will allow you to experience the basic concept of meditation. You'll get a glimmer of how pleasant it is to shut off the countless thoughts that are constantly flying around in your head, in order to savor a few moments of peace and quiet.

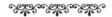

Personal Anecdote:
Do Not Disturb: Meditation in Progress

Looking for a calm place that was free of distractions, which in my house is like looking for a zoo without animals, I decided to meditate in a large walk-in closet. I didn't tell my kids what I was up to, figuring that if I left a few dollars on the kitchen counter, I could disappear for twenty minutes without being missed. I knew that if I told them what I was doing they'd be convinced that I was one sandwich short of a picnic and add it to their arsenal when they played, "my mother is crazier than yours" with their friends.

As luck would have it, as I was in the middle of a meditation, one of my daughters decided to come over and search the house for an article of clothing that she hadn't worn in five years. Not realizing that I was sitting on the floor of the closet, she flung open the door, bumped into me and screamed, nearly giving us both heart attacks. Thoughtful soul that she is, the next time she caught me in the closet, she hung a sign on the door that read, "Do not disturb. Meditation in progress." The moral of this story: If you decide to meditate, instruct other people not to bug you while you're doing it. At the very least, you'll have some time to yourself.

Progressive muscle relaxation

This is a technique in which you focus on the tension in a particular muscle group and then consciously release it. You can even use it to help you fall asleep at night, assuming that nothing better comes up.

As with meditation, find a quiet place away from distractions and get into a comfortable position. I prefer to be reclining. Take several deep breaths, trying to get rid of stress as you exhale. Starting with your feet, tighten the muscles as hard as you can, hold the tension in them for a few seconds, then let them go limp. Gradually move up your entire body the same way—lower legs, knees, thighs, buttocks, hips, abdominals, chest, back, shoulders, arms, neck, and finally your face and scalp. If you haven't relaxed by the time you get to the top of your head, go back to your feet and start all over again.

DEEP BREATHING

What could possibly be more practical than using deep, slow breathing to calm yourself down? Whether you use it alone or in conjunction with progressive relaxation, it brings extra oxygen to the brain, decreases your blood pressure, slows your pulse rate, and relaxes tense muscles. You can do it anywhere, anytime that you feel tension mounting.

Try it next time you're in a long line at the bank and all of the tellers go on break. To get started, breathe in through your nose for a slow count of four, hold it for four, then exhale through your mouth for four. When this is comfortable for you, increase the count to eight.

You can also try deep abdominal or diaphragmatic breathing, a more advanced technique often used in yoga, but save this one for when you're alone. As you inhale very slowly through your nose, allow your diaphragm to contract and your stomach and chest to expand. Reverse as you exhale through your mouth. You can tell if you're doing it properly by placing your hands on your abdomen, right above the navel. Your hands should rise as you inhale and fall as you exhale.

JUST FOR RELAXATION

I have four suggestions for stress relief that are not exercise related but that will definitely contribute to your health and well-being. After all, part of being fit is the ability to relax.

MASSAGE

Sometimes all it takes is a little pampering to relieve stress. Massages are a perfect way to let go.

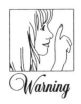

Warning

If you're looking for a restful massage, the type where your body turns into liquid and slides off the table, avoid any of the deep-tissue varieties such as shiatsu or rolfing. Although these will definitely get the kinks out of your muscles, they're often painful and are usually administered by ex-prison matrons who were forced into early retirement.

115

Aromatherapy

For most people, there is a strong link between mood and fragrance. Aromatherapy uses this link to create pleasant sensations and emotional responses that will restore your mind and body. All you have to do is find a scented oil that you like, put a few drops in the bath or even on your arm, close your eyes and let the aroma take over. What I think might be even more effective is to find out what type of cologne Robert Redford wears, splash a little of that around the tub, close your eyes and pretend he's in there with you.

Visualization

In the tub or elsewhere, visualization is the act of using your imagination to take a short vacation from stress. Sit back, close your eyes and picture yourself in the most beautiful, serene setting that you can possibly envision. (Whom, if anyone, you'd like to place in the setting with you is entirely up to your discretion.) Keep the picture in your mind until a calming sensation takes over.

Special places

A simple way to relieve stress is to find a readily accessible place that comforts you, and to spend a little time there as often as possible. I'm not referring to four-star hotels, which I happen to find very comforting, but rather to places in nature. Don't worry, this doesn't mean that you have to go camping or anything as threatening as that. I'm merely suggesting that you take a walk on the beach, watch the sunset from a favorite hill, or sit in a garden.

A FINAL NOTE ON STRESS

Stress is always going to be around in one form or another. It's important to learn how to control it, instead of letting it control you. Since there are so many pleasant ways to do that, you just might miss it if it was gone. The next time you're getting a massage, soaking in a bubble bath, or visualizing yourself in Tahiti, remember that stress is an ideal reason to call time out.

Chapter 11

Help!
Where Do I Begin?

DO I REALLY HAVE TO DO IT ALL?

Now that I've clued you in as to what it takes to get in shape (sensible nutrition, cardiovascular exercise, weight training, stretching, and stress management), you're probably asking yourself, "Does she really expect me to do all of that? Is she on drugs?" Take heart, you're not a total fitness failure if you omit one of the elements. It's just that you're cheating yourself out of the healthiest, most attractive body that you could possibly have. (Can you tell from that guilt trip that I've been a mother for many years?) Remember, we do it because we're desperate, and desperate women can't afford to cut corners.

LOOK, MA—SCIENTIFIC EVIDENCE

If you don't want to take my word for it, consider some scientific evidence. James M. Rippe, a cardiologist and fitness researcher at the University of Massachusetts Medical School, did a study that confirmed the importance of a well-rounded program in terms of weight loss and body composition. He demonstrated that dieters who did aerobics and weight training, not only lost more weight, they increased their percentage of lean body mass, improving their muscle to fat ratio.

Whether or not you're trying to lose weight, it's important to increase your muscle to fat ratio with proper nutrition and exercise because excess fat puts an unnecessary burden on your heart, lungs, kidney, and liver. It can also diminish your energy, your enthusiasm, and your wardrobe choices.

Furthermore, muscle tissue is metabolically more active (burns more calories) than flab. This means that a 130 pound lean person can eat more calories per day than a 130 pound fat person. Now doesn't that give you incentive? Another thought to keep in mind is that most mature adults who don't exercise lose about a half pound of muscle a year.

Although it is generally acknowledged that cardiovascular fitness is essential to health, the concept of a complete fitness package is becoming more widely accepted. Dr. Kenneth Cooper, author of *Aerobics,* states: "Aerobics are merely the foundation for a good exercise program."

The American College of Sports Medicine, the leading organization in sports medicine and exercise science, recommends aerobic exercise three to five times per week for twenty to sixty minutes (preferably four to five times per week for at least thirty minutes if your main objective is weight loss), and strength training two or three times per week. As for stretching, once you're warmed up, you should do it before, during, and after your workout.

KEEPING THE MACHINE RUNNING

The analogy of the body as a machine, which I used to emphasize the importance of stretching, also illustrates the need for an overall commitment to staying fit and healthy. Think of your body as an incredible and priceless machine with a lot of extremely complicated parts. If those parts get rusty and break down, then the whole machine breaks down. And believe me, it's not that easy to repair, so you're better off keeping it well-tuned and running. If you're still not convinced, picture yourself having to wear a muumuu for the rest of your life!

WHERE DO I START?

Let's assume that my powers of persuasion have won you over, and you're ready to take the plunge. You're just not quite sure how to plan a program that's going to work for you—one that satisfies your needs, keeps you interested, and gives you the best results.

A simple method for developing your routine is to approach the task like a tabloid journalist. Determine the who, what, where, when, why, and how of your exercise regime by answering the following personal questions.

(Despite the suggestive nature of the questions, they are not about sex. If, however, you can work up enough enthusiasm to sustain high energy sex for at least twenty minutes, you can include it as part of your cardiovascular workout).

What would you most enjoy doing?

No matter how much you may hate to work out, you still have to do it, so at least look for something that you find less objectionable. Before jumping on any exercise bandwagon, take the time to consider your likes and dislikes, your strengths and weaknesses.

Let's assume that you're allergic to being outdoors and can't find your way to the bathroom in the middle of the night. You can safely rule out hiking and backpacking as two of your top choices. If you're afraid of water, don't like to blow dry your hair, and would rather die than be seen in public without makeup, swimming and scuba diving should not be high on your list of options. I must say though, synchronized swimmers have cute waterproof caps and some sort of makeup that stays on forever, so if you could get over your fear of the water, you might be okay.

You also have to face the fact that some activities are simply not for everyone because they're more difficult to master and require a greater level of natural skill. However, if you feel that you were born to fence, take a stab at it before settling on something easier. You might be surprised at what you can accomplish with a combination of desire, determination, and desperation.

With **whom** would you like to do it?

In selecting a sport or activity, you have to take into account the number of people that you'll need to do it. You may love to play softball, yet it's not always easy to round up a team. I know a woman who was a softball fanatic, but her husband got suspicious when she kept playing until two in the morning. He couldn't believe that she could find a lit field at that hour, let alone an umpire and seventeen other players.

Working out alone has the advantage of letting you go whenever you have the time, but it's often tough to find the motivation. The buddy system is an excellent alternative because you only have to rely on one other person. It also forces you to show up unless you want to invent one dumb excuse after another about why you couldn't be there.

Warning

Be wary of partners who have more lame excuses than you do. In case you're not sure, "I can't jog today because I have a broken leg," is a legitimate excuse. "I can't jog because I have a broken nail," isn't. Also watch out for training partners who fake injuries. On the broken leg, I might ask to see the cast.

Try to find someone whose personality and workout style are compatible with your own. If you're more laid back and methodical, don't invite trouble by trying to

train with someone who acts as if she's overdosed on hor-
mones. If you're not competitive, don't hook up with
someone who goes for the world sit-up record every time
she hits the floor.

When would you like to do it?

There are no hard and fast rules as to what time you have to exercise, and there are even a few health clubs that stay open twenty-four hours a day. If possible, try working out at different hours to see when you feel your best. Do you have more energy in the morning or does it take you until noon to get into gear? Will hitting the gym after dinner insure a sound night's sleep or keep you awake until dawn?

Some scientists believe that there is a set of biorhythms called circadian rhythms which occurs every twenty-four hours. Circadian rhythms are based on a day-night cycle, with these cycles broken into periods of activity and periods of rest. Although it's generally accepted that certain creatures such as bats, owls, and mothers of newborns are nocturnal, most people are more active during the day. You may, however, be one of those women who doesn't fit the mold.

If you're a night person, you'll be more productive if you can some-how accommodate your propensity to be active after dark. You don't have to give up your day job and turn to bartending, but you might arrange your schedule so that you can stay up later at night and get some extra sleep in the morning.

Where would you like to do it?

If you're so disgustingly well-adjusted and gung ho that you can do aerobics in front of a small-screen, black and white TV in your own liv-ing room, you probably don't understand the significance of this ques-tion. As for those of you who get physically ill if you even think about exercising at home and who use every phone call as an excuse to take a break, it's essential to find a place that's convenient, comfortable, and compatible with your needs. (See section entitled "Selecting a Health Club.")

There are some activities, such as walking, that you can do almost any time and any place, while others will require special equipment and facilities. If you find yourself drawn to the latter, check into the expense before you get too involved. Also take into account the climate where you live. If the weather's pleasant, why not exercise outdoors to take advantage of it?

How do you want to look while you're doing it?

Another key factor in choosing the form of self-abuse, oops, I mean the form of exercise that's best for you, is the outfit. To paraphrase the old saying, "It's not whether you win or lose, it's how you look while you're playing the game." Do you really think that tennis would be as popular if the outfits weren't so cute? Do you know why more women don't play basketball or soccer? Bad shorts. With a bit less violence, I think that football could become the wave of the future because the shoulder pads and the tight pants are a great look. The helmets need some rethinking, but on a bad hair day, they work.

You should also check out the bodies and facial expressions of women who've been involved in the activity for awhile. Take marathon runners, for instance. They're usually skinny, which may appeal to you, but how many of them have you ever seen smiling when they're on the road. Ditto for long distance bike riders, but at least they have fabulous calves, and they get to sit down while they're working out. I've always had fantasies about becoming a beach volleyball player. They've got beautiful tans, nice bodies, and big smiles because they know how terrific they look.

Why do I even have to do this in first place?

Come on, you know the answer to this one. It's the big "D". It's desperation! If you don't want to turn into a crumbling, old-for-her-age crone with no energy and a bad attitude, you've got to get with the program. You've got to exercise, eat right, and take better care of yourself. Let desperation give you the incentive to transform yourself from a thrift shop special to a well-preserved antique.

Chapter 12

The Health Club: Your Home Away from Home

Personal Anecdote: Selecting a Health Club

As a novice exerciser, I joined a plush health club that had lovely forest green carpeting, shiny chrome weights, deodorant and hair spray in the locker room, and showers without visible signs of mildew. The club also offered valet parking, a beauty salon, and a restaurant. After spending so much time there that I had just about decided to leave my family and move in, I experienced a shocking revelation. I needed more, or less, depending on your perspective. I had turned into a hard core weight lifter who wanted to pump iron, not chrome.

Not sure what to expect, I dragged a friend along for moral support and joined a muscle gym. Talk about culture shock, it was like walking into the black hole. I had the urge to hang curtains, bring in plants, and spray disinfectant. I never found out if the showers were moldy because I was afraid to go into the locker room. The fitness floor was filled with huge people with hairy chests and bulging muscles—and the men were even worse. I hadn't seen so much sweat or heard so much grunting since I'd been in labor.

Despite my initial reservations, I kept going back until I enjoyed the smell and could pick up heavy weights without falling on the floor. Eventually, I grew to love that place. I became friends with people named "Butch" and "Bubba." I even stopped calling the women "sir." I became such a regular that the other members quit making fun of me for wearing perfume, makeup, and earrings when I worked out.

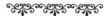

The point is, you have to find a health club that "fits." If you're truly desperate, the place that you work out is going to be your home away from home so you'd better make sure that it's right for you. It's like investing in a timeshare condo except that all of the owners share it simultaneously.

TYPES OF CLUBS

There are many different types of clubs, each one with a unique personality. From hard core to deluxe, from family fitness centers to yuppie gathering places, from women only to anyone welcome who can pay the dues—there's something for everyone. Take your own peculiarities and preferences into account and visit several before making a commitment.

If your near-sighted beloved is the only man allowed to view you in a leotard, you'll be much happier at a women only club. To the contrary, if men inspire you to new heights of performance, or if you're searching for someone to keep you in your old age, an upscale, co-ed venue is definitely for you. Although you can learn to work out anywhere, being in the right place is its own form of motivation.

WHAT TO LOOK FOR

When researching a health club, arrange your visit for the time of day that you intend to use it. Tour the facilities, or better yet, find out if there is a complimentary visit for potential members so that you can test the equipment, talk to the staff, and get a feel for the atmosphere. Keep the following factors in mind when making your decision.

LOCATION

First and foremost is location. If a club isn't close to your home or office, you won't use it as often as you should, no matter how wonderful it may be. It also helps if the club is in a safe area so that you won't be afraid of getting mugged every time you walk out the front door. If the neighborhood is less than desirable, ask about security.

PARKING

Be sure there's adequate and convenient parking, especially if you're going to be there during peak hours. When you're searching for a reason to dodge your workout, trouble with parking may be all it takes to send you on your merry way. If there's one thing you don't need, it's another excuse.

THE FACILITY

You can tell a lot about a health club simply by walking around the facility. Is it clean? Is it well-maintained? Is the atmosphere friendly? Are the exercise and class areas bright, roomy, and well-ventilated, or are they dark, overcrowded dungeons?

Don't overlook the locker room because you may be spending more time there than you realize. Locker rooms run the gamut from plush retreats that you wouldn't mind having in your own home, to those that resemble something out of a downtown bus station. The worst setup I ever encountered was a co-ed arrangement at a hard-core gym. Forget about changing your clothes. If you needed to use the bathroom, you had to shout from the doorway to be sure there weren't any naked men strutting around.

By glancing at bulletin boards and posters you can get an idea of the events and services that are available. You can also discern if the club is more concerned with social activities or if the emphasis is on fitness and health.

MEMBERSHIP

If your tour of a health club is followed by some fast talking gorilla trying to convince you to sign a lifetime contract in blood, turn around and run! The same holds true if a membership person seems more desperate than you are and calls you so often that you have to get an unlisted number.

Most health clubs charge a one time initiation fee and monthly dues, although some may discount the amount if you pay annually. Many places run frequent specials when they waive the initiation fee or offer reduced rate, trial memberships. Some will even allow you to join for non-prime time hours at a lower rate or give you a special deal if you join at the recommendation of a member.

Don't pay more than you can afford and be sure that you're getting your money's worth. Some of the more expensive fitness centers provide fancy newsletters, social events, lectures, and other fringe benefits. If you don't care about these extras or if they're not in your budget, find a place that caters strictly to your exercise needs.

EXTRAS

Be specific as to what's included in your membership. Find out if personal training is provided or if it's available at a discounted rate. (The cost of personal training varies from state to state and even from club to club.) Ask if all classes are included or if some require additional fees. Some clubs will charge for classes such as martial arts or dance which may be taught by non-staff instructors. See if nutritional counseling is part of the membership package or if it's another extra.

EQUIPMENT AND CLASSES

Check to see that the fitness center has adequate equipment for the number of people who are using it and that the equipment is well cared for. Two bad omens are lines of people taking numbers to get on machines, and "sorry, out of order" signs posted on every other piece of equipment.

Request a class schedule to find out what's offered and when. Inquire as to class sizes and level of difficulty.

STAFF

The staff of a club should be knowledgeable, readily available, and pleasant. Notice if the staff members are assisting people, offering encouragement and advice, or just standing around and flexing. Find out if they're certified by one of the fitness organizations such as ACSM, ACE, or AFAA.

Ask if the staff will provide an initial fitness screening, set you up on a program, and monitor your progress. Find out if they provide a written record so that you can eventually keep track of your own workouts.

If you're really age or appearance sensitive, be certain there's someone who will be sympathetic to your needs. Not every instructor has to look as if she just stepped off the cover of a health magazine to have the expertise that you need. You might want to inquire as to the specific exercise background of various instructors.

MEMBERS

Call me shallow again, but I think you should check out the members to see if they're people you'd like to exercise with. Sweating together in revealing clothing is pretty personal and not something you'd like to do with just anyone.

Furthermore, it'll help your workouts to be around people whose goals are similar to your own and who have to work as hard as you do to stay in shape. You don't necessarily have to avoid young, gorgeous women with perfect bodies, but wouldn't it be nice to exercise with someone that you didn't want to kill?

The Health Club Etiquette Quiz

Many older women are intimidated by the mere thought of joining a health club. Aside from being self-conscious about their physical condition, they worry about being placed in unfamiliar and potentially embarrassing situations. Have no fear, take this quiz and you'll be saved from making your share of gym faux pas.

Q: What do you do if you're waiting for a machine and the sweat monster who's using it gets up and walks away without wiping the seat?

A: You have four choices:
   a. Use your own towel to wipe off the machine.
   b. Sit down and try to ignore the sweat.
   c. Skip the machine entirely.
   d. Request that the offender come back and clean up.

I suggest that you go with option d. If the offender isn't cooperative, you'll at least be getting a valuable lesson in assertiveness training.

Q: What do you do if you're waiting to use a piece of equipment and the person on the machine is doing multiple sets?

A: It's perfectly acceptable to ask "May I work in with you?" or "How many sets do you have left?" The usual reply will be, "Of course," or "I just have one set left, and then it's all yours." If you get an attitude from someone, this is probably the same type of person who leaves sweat on the machines and not someone you'd want to work in with anyway.

Q: What do you do if someone gets off a machine without unloading the weights, or leaves dumbbells on the floor?

A: You can:
   a. Confront him if you have the nerve or tell an employee if you don't.
   b. Ignore the situation and suffer in silence.

The recommendation is for a. It's not your job to pick up after people in the gym, no matter how many children you may have.

Q: Should you fake it if you don't know how to use a machine?

A: Faking it is never a good idea, if you get my drift. You won't enjoy the benefits of the exercise and may even hurt yourself. Ask for assistance.

Q: Is it okay to wear makeup when you work out? What about perfume?
A: Do I even have to answer the first part of this question.

Makeup is mandatory. (See section titled "illusion.") As for perfume, keep it to a minimum. The scent gets stronger as you sweat and can become offensive or cause allergy problems for other people.

Q: Are all locker room scales five pounds too high?

A: Judging from the comments I've heard—absolutely!

Q: What do you do if someone corrects you or offers unsolicited advice while you're working out?

A: There are two different responses depending on whether the person is male or female.
   a. If it's a female, before you get defensive and snap "no, thank-

you," consider the source and see if you'd like your body to be more like hers. If not, look her up and down and then chuckle to yourself.

b. If it's a male who's sharing his wisdom, figure out his motives. If he's cute enough and you're interested enough, you may have to listen to some stupid advice.

Q: What do you do if a younger person in the gym calls you "ma'am"?

A: Use your seniority to have that person kicked out of the health club.

Chapter 13

Mistakes

COMMON MISTAKES AND HOW TO AVOID THEM

There are some common mistakes that can sabotage even the most well thought out fitness program. Although these mistakes are more frequently committed by novices, not even seasoned exercise queens are immune. They are:

- Enrolling in an exercise class taught by a twenty year old named Bubbles; actually by anyone named Bubbles
- Wearing a leotard that's one size too small
- Neglecting to check for sweat before sitting down on a machine

Aside from these typical errors, there are four more that can do even more serious damage, making the difference between your success or failure.

MISTAKE #1—BEING INCONSISTENT AND DISORGANIZED

If you take a catch-as-catch-can approach to exercise and throw in a sit-up here and a sit-up there, your body is never going to respond the way that you want it to. You can't just do your workouts when the mood strikes or when you have nothing better to do. You have to schedule them into your daily routine if you expect to see results.

Whether you believe the hype that you can do it all in twenty minutes three times a week (give me a break, it takes longer than that to get ready to exercise), or whether you intend to spend several hours, you should have a plan for each session as well as a general plan for the week.

The Fitness Journal

The most practical way to keep track of your aerobics, weight training, stretching, and nutrition is to set up a fitness journal or notebook. Some gyms may provide them for you.

Originally I started keeping a journal because I couldn't remember what I was doing from one day to the next. On Tuesday I couldn't even tell you if I'd been to the gym on Monday, let alone which body parts I'd worked. Writing it down let me see what I had accomplished and what I needed to do next. It put my whole routine in context.

Aside from using a journal to organize and schedule your workouts, you can use it to chart your progress. Keep a record of specific weight training exercises along with sets, reps, and poundage to validate improvements in strength and endurance. Write down the type of aerobic work that you do, including duration of the exercise and your maximum heart rate. Also note any increase in flexibility.

Depending on how detailed you make your observations, a journal can enable you to recognize how other factors such as eating habits and anxiety are influencing your overall effectiveness. Jotting down information about your nutrition, performance, and moods also enables you to stay in touch with your natural cycles or biorhythms and to work **with** your body instead of against it. Just don't stress out if you forget to write anything down for a day or two; this is a personal account for your own benefit, not your parole board hearing.

A sample entry might contain a brief record of your workout along with comments such as, "Did 500 sit-ups today because I was bloated and felt like a pig. Throw out pink leotard and tights," or "I'm incredible. Did an hour on the treadmill without needing three cups of coffee. Time to give up caffeine?"

Although there are ready-made journals on the market, all you really need is an inexpensive notebook, datebook, or calendar. I used to write things down on deposit slips, toilet paper, gas receipts, or whatever else was handy and then throw them in my gym bag, but I wouldn't recommend that approach. After awhile your gym bag will look like a trash can, and you'll still be totally disorganized.

MISTAKE #2—SETTING UNREALISTIC GOALS

Setting goals is an excellent exercise strategy, but setting goals that are well beyond your wildest dreams is the quickest way to get discouraged. The trick is to simplify, to start with the minimum and gradually increase the difficulty of your routine and the level of your expectations. Set up short term goals that are well within reach and long term goals that are more demanding but still feasible. Accomplishing the short term will serve as periodic reinforcement on your way to the biggie.

For instance, if you're really out of shape, your long term goal may be to get through an advanced aerobics class without needing oxygen. Your short range goals may be to complete half of a beginning class within two weeks, the entire class within four, and an intermediate class within two months. If you're trying to shed thirty pounds, focus on losing a pound or two a week instead of thinking about all thirty. If you'd eventually like to run a marathon, first train for a 5K and then a 10K.

Mistake #3—Overtraining

Overtraining puts excess wear and tear on your body and makes you susceptible to injury and exhaustion. It can be a matter of exercising too often or trying to do too much within each session. If you find yourself packed in ice after every workout or wearing more Ace bandages than clothing, your body is definitely showing signs of overuse.

Although everyone should avoid overtraining, in some ways it's even more important for novices and those of you on the comeback trail. Striving to make up for lost time, you may be tempted to overdo your entire exercise regimen, but this is a huge mistake. Instead of feeling fired up and energized, you'll soon be exhausted and sore because your body won't be able to keep up with your enthusiasm. You may be a real dynamo for awhile, but it won't last.

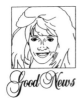

If you take some time off after exercising regularly for years, the decline is even slower and less severe. It's like the difference between a building that's been renovated and just requires regular upkeep and a dilapidated eyesore that needs a lot of work.

Start out with the minimum recommendation of three to five, twenty to thirty minute periods of aerobic activity per week, along with two or three short sessions of strength building, and some gentle stretching, either on its own or incorporated into your other exercise. As you progress, increase the duration, the frequency, or the intensity of your workouts.

I've seen countless desperate women trying to get in shape by working out eight days a week. When I'd caution them about what they were doing, they'd claim to be different, to enjoy living at the health club, and to feel no remorse at abandoning their friends and loved ones. But no matter how sincere these women sounded, I never saw one who lasted for more than a few months before disappearing forever. I have no idea where they all went, but I have a strong suspicion that they became members of a cult that practices sunbathing, donut worship, and shopping.

Remember, staying fit is a lifetime commitment, not something that you do over a long weekend. Give your body a chance. It took you a long time to get out of shape, and it's going to take you a long time to get back in, but don't get discouraged. Compared to the early hurdles, maintenance is a snap.

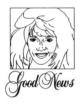 *Those of you who are dedicated, long-term exercisers needn't panic if you have to take a short break. You can safely take off a week or two without losing much ground and may actually be giving your hard working body a sorely needed rest. Even if you goof off a bit longer than two weeks, you can usually regain your level of fitness in a relatively short time.*

MISTAKE #4—GETTING STUCK IN A RUT

Doing the same thing every time you worked out would be like serving the exact same meal for dinner every night. No matter how delicious it tasted, after awhile you'd be so sick and tired of it, you wouldn't even want to pick up the phone to order it.

When you first begin training it's helpful to stick with a basic routine until you're comfortable with the movements and familiar with what you're doing. Once that happens, it's time to move on or you'll get stuck in such a deep rut that you'll die of boredom before you die of old age.

Cross-training, varying the type of exercise that you do from day to day or week to week, will not only alleviate that boredom but will also prevent injury by allowing you to work different muscle groups and avoid overuse of the same body parts. You can vary your whole fitness routine—walking one day, weight lifting the next, bicycling the day after that—or you can try different forms of what you're already used to. If you've been taking the same stretch class every week for six months, change instructors or switch over to yoga. If you've been using weight training machines, take the plunge and experiment with free weights. If the seat of the Lifecycle is imprinted with your rear end, try the treadmill instead.

Recreational sports can also be used to add some spice to your life. They may not get your heart rate up and keep it within your training zone, but they're usually more exciting than say, swimming 400 laps or running five miles. According to Doug Miller, a fitness researcher at the University of Tennessee at Memphis, "Recreational sports also complement aerobic activities because they involve intense bursts of muscle activity." These bursts provide anaerobic conditioning which forces the muscles to react quickly and may also improve your agility and coordination.

❧❧❧

PERSONAL ANECDOTE:
HOW I MADE EVERY MISTAKE IN THE BOOK PLUS A FEW EXTRAS

(This section is purely anecdotal so you have every right to skip it, but I think you'd be making a big mistake.)

As you may have guessed, I have first hand familiarity with all of these mistakes, but I overcame them and so can you. It just takes a measure of common sense and a large helping of persistence.

Having spent most of my life as a devout non–athlete and never having participated in a competitive sport, I was not a likely exercise candidate. I dabbled a bit in my childbearing years because I was having nightmares about my body—one night I dreamt that it exploded— but I never really took it too seriously. (How can you take anything seriously when you have three kids?)

When I finally took the plunge, I was so eager to get into shape and so clueless about what I was doing, that I made every mistake in the book (plus a few others that weren't in there). For starters, I accepted advice from anyone with a persuasive manner. If the health club janitor was the least bit convincing when he told me that I wasn't working with enough weight, I increased the poundage. If someone in decent shape told me that her secret was aerobics or running or jumping, I tried it. On one occasion, on the advice of some lunatic with great legs, I hopped up and down bleachers like a frog. I'm lucky that I'm still alive and have knees.

Another mistake I made was not taking notes when an instructor at the health club took me through my first routine. It didn't seem to be all that complicated when he led me from machine to machine and told me exactly what to do. Besides, I couldn't stop staring at his biceps which were the size of large grapefruits. I went through the motions and then collected the card where he'd written down the basics of what he'd shown me. When he offered to make an appointment to go through it again on my next visit, I assured him that wouldn't be necessary. I was certain that I could figure it out on my own.

When I came in to work out by myself a few days later, it was a disaster. I couldn't remember which machine worked what, how the seats were supposed to be adjusted, how I was supposed to sit, how I was supposed to breathe, or what I was doing there in the first place. I was also convinced that everyone was staring at me. Too embarrassed to ask for help, I tried to sneak out a side door, but set off the emergency alarm.

About two weeks later, when I finally gathered up the courage to return, I considered a disguise, but instead pretended that I'd never been there before. This time I came prepared. I took notes, drew diagrams, spoke into a tape recorder, and photographed other people using the equipment. Despite all that back-up, it still took me six months before I really felt comfortable. (I don't even want to know what the trainers thought about me.) To this day, I get intimidated if I go to a gym that has complicated looking apparatus. If a sign explaining the use of a machine has more than one paragraph—forget it.

My initial experience with free weights is another perfect example of my bumbling. Although I was never really too enthralled with weight training machines, I stuck with them for ages because I was afraid to make a change. But from the moment I picked up my first dumbbell, I was hooked. As a result, I did far too many exercises, forgetting that this was something entirely new for my body and might make me sore. Let me tell you, sore didn't come close to describing the way that I felt the next morning. Run over by a truck was more like it.

I had my first hint of what was to come when I went into the locker room after working out. I tried to pick up my hairbrush, but my arms were shaking so badly, it took three attempts before I got it into my hand. Then I hit myself in the face with it. Since I couldn't zip my pants, button my shirt, or tie my shoes, I didn't know whether to spend the night in the locker room or wrap myself in a towel and crawl to the car. (Walking wasn't an option because my legs were in spasm.) After begging someone for a ride home, I fell into bed and slept for twelve hours.

Was I in for a surprise when I woke up the next morning. I never hop out of bed, but I can usually manage to hit the floor in an upright position and stagger to the bathroom. Not that day. When I hit the floor, it was in a sprawl. An hour later, when I made it to the bathroom, I was thankful that I kept so much reading material in there because once I sat down, there was no way that I could get right back up. It took me three days, not to get out of the bathroom, but to feel as if my body had returned to almost normal.

Even after that experience, I had a tendency to weight lift to exhaustion. I'd come home from the gym and feel as if I'd spent the day working construction. I also had an appetite like a construction worker and atrocious eating habits. If my metabolism hadn't been working overtime, I'd probably have become a candidate for the first American female sumo wrestler.

As for a well-rounded, organized program, words like "cardiovascular" and "aerobic" weren't in my vocabulary, let alone in my life. When someone who was coaching me in weight lifting suggested that I run or ride a bike, I suggested that he get psychiatric counseling.

Instead of alleviating stress, my routine was creating it. Between three children and a husband who was more a fan of dinner on the table than of bodybuilding (He's come a long way, baby!), I was going crazy trying to sneak in my hours at the health club. When I was home, I wanted to be at the gym. When I was working out, I felt as if I should be home with my family. I knew I was in trouble when I began curling frying pans and bench pressing my kids. It was around the same time that I started yelling at people in the gym to pick up their weights and behave themselves. I think the only thing that would have solved my dilemma was a new identity, like a witness protection program for *overwrought women who've suddenly decided to become athletes.*

To this day I have problems fitting it all in, but I don't let it bother me as much, which goes a long way toward stress reduction. I've also convinced my husband and daughters that the family that trains together, remains together. Well, I tried to convince them. Unfortunately, they were laughing so hard they almost choked on their Twinkies. When they calmed down, they all agreed to go to the gym if I promised never to say anything like that to them again.

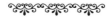

Chapter 14

Motivation

INITIAL MOTIVATION

Your initial impetus for shaping up may come from many different sources—photos of yourself in a bathing suit taken without your prior knowledge or consent, catty comments from so-called friends about the size of your derriere, the sight of your husband drooling over the latest *Sports Illustrated* swimsuit edition. Although effective, these forms of incentive are usually temporary.

The challenge is to stay with a program long enough to develop the inner drive or impulse which will make it virtually impossible for you to stop exercising and eating right, even if you want to. The word "inner" is the key because despite what opinions, advice, or encouragement other people may offer, they're not going to do the work for you. You're the only one who can get the job done.

Over the years I've spoken to countless long-term exercisers about what it takes to stay motivated. From their comments and from my own experience I can assure you, aside from this inner drive which is born out of long habit plus a measure of desperation, we each have a few tricks up our sleeves that keep us going when good intentions fail. The following techniques are guaranteed to help you stick with a program whether you've been around the exercise block a few times or are just about to begin.

HANDY MOTIVATIONAL TECHNIQUES

VISUALIZE

Visualization, an effective tool for relaxation, can also be used for motivation. To mentally prepare for a workout session, picture yourself in action, focused and confident, with the body of your youth. Remind yourself that the exercise you're about to do will bring you one step closer to reclaiming that body.

You can also use visualization to energize yourself. During exercise, particularly weight lifting, imagine a colored light (I prefer purple) carrying bursts of power to your muscles. You can do this with music too. When you're on a treadmill or stationary bike listening to music, imagine the sounds traveling throughout your body like currents of energy. If that doesn't work, close your eyes and pretend that you're somewhere else doing something illegal or fattening.

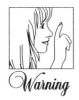

When listening to music on a headset, try not to sing along because you won't realize how loud your voice is. I mention this because despite being so tone deaf that I generally restrict my performances to the shower or the car, when I put on a headset, I have an unfortunate tendency to belt out songs as if I'm in concert. I didn't realize quite how awful I sounded until someone, who thought I was dying, called the paramedics.

FANTASIZE

I was explaining the concept of picturing yourself to be somewhere else to a friend who hates to exercise, when she suddenly exclaimed, "I know exactly what you mean! Fantasize!" We immediately agreed that any woman over forty who says that she doesn't have a rich fantasy life is either lying, misinformed, or dating young boys. We have to use this to our advantage.

I don't know what kind of tapes my non-exercising friend bought for her Walkman or where she was imagining herself to be, but the last time I saw her she was on a treadmill, decked out in a pink leotard with lace tights. She had lost twenty pounds and couldn't stop smiling.

Curious about the type of fantasies that other women were using to keep themselves motivated, I started asking around and got some interesting answers. A woman on the rowing machine said that she often imagines herself on a Coast Guard rescue mission. Another, a frustrated actress, pictures an audience at her workouts. The problem is that she wastes a lot of time waiting for applause. Still another stays on the treadmill by pretending that she's being chased by muggers! After hearing that, I decided that perhaps I was learning more than I ever really wanted to know about other women in the gym.

FIND SOME DIVERSION

There are people who would disagree with what I'm about to suggest (So what else is new?), claiming that it diminishes your intensity, but I contend that sometimes you have to make tradeoffs. What I'm referring to is entertaining yourself when you're on a piece of cardiovascular equipment. If you have a short attention span and are easily bored, there's no way that you're going to stay on a stairmaster or bike for any length of time unless you have something else to keep you amused.

Simultaneously watching TV, listening to tapes, and reading a book works for me. I've even tried dancing at the same time that I was using the equipment, but this is tricky on treadmills and steps, and nearly impossible on a bike or rowing machine unless you stand on the seat. Granted, you may sacrifice some intensity by scattering your concentration, but at least you'll be extending the duration of your workout. And as you recall, a fat-burning workout is lower in intensity and longer in duration.

Here's an interesting diversion to use when someone stops by your machine to chat. Rate her personality on a scale of one to ten by the amount of time that elapses without your realizing it. If you think that someone's been talking to you for at least twenty minutes and then glance at your readout and see that only two minutes have gone by, score her a one and cut the conversation short. You're better off with a Walkman. If someone is so amusing that the minutes seem to fly by, score her a ten and try to keep her talking for as long as possible.

If you're not in the mood for company, put on your earphones, even if the tape is off, shut your eyes and pretend that you're engrossed in whatever you're supposed to be doing. If someone still insists on bothering you, roll up your towel and snap it at her!

Never keep your eyes on the digital time readout on an exercise machine or you'll gain new insight into the expression, "time stood still." As soon as you get started, cover the numbers with a towel. Hope that when you peek at them again, you'll be thrilled to see how many minutes have gone by.

Use Flash Cards

Students use flash cards to help recall material that they're studying. You can use flash cards to help recall the reasons that you have to exercise. You can use scare tactics and write down words such as "cellulite," "high blood pressure," "desperation" and "fat." Or go with something more positive and write down the wonderful results you can expect such as "stronger muscles," "longer life," and "fewer doctor bills." Place the cards in strategic locations (the refrigerator, dashboard, bathroom mirror) as constant reminders. If you need an extra push, gather them in a pile and read them over and over before you fall asleep at night.

USE MANTRAS

Using a mantra is similar to using flash cards in that repetition is important. The difference is that you repeat one or two choice phrases over and over in your head. What you say is up to you, but here are some suggestions:

- I exercise because I'm desperate.
- Lifting weights will keep me from looking like a large Jell-O mold.
- I'm going to be the strongest woman in the retirement home.
- I'm not my mother.
- I love endorphins.
- Only fifty more years and I can stop doing this.

LOOK IN THE MIRROR (NOT FOR THE FAINTHEARTED)

Once a week get naked and observe yourself in a mirror. If you stick with your program, you will eventually be able to do this without needing a stiff drink. If you slack off, one glance should get you back on track.

PLAY MIND GAMES

Another way to keep going is to play psychological games with yourself. In an aerobics class, for example, pinpoint someone who seems to be in slightly better condition than you are. Label her the enemy and then refuse to quit until she breaks down. Or promise yourself that if you can make it to the end of a class without passing out or in some other way embarrassing yourself, that you'll never have to do it again. I know a woman who loathes aerobics but gets through three classes a week by using this method.

You can also trick your body into longer workouts by setting continuous short range goals. Perhaps tell yourself that you only have to keep hiking until you reach a certain tree. Once you've reached it, select a new point and so on.

REWARD YOURSELF

Reward yourself for performing at a certain level or for a specified period of time. If you stick with a program for a month, buy yourself a new outfit. If you complete three weight training sessions, go for a massage. On a smaller scale, reward yourself for twenty minutes of cardiovascular exercise with a bottle of non-carbonated mineral water. This last one may not sound like much, but when you're thirsty, you'll feel as if you're drinking champagne.

Along the same lines, add something that you enjoy to your workout experience. Read a trashy novel while you're on the bike, window shop while you're walking, or treat yourself to some new tapes. This is especially important if you know that you're always going to regard exercise as a nuisance or a chore. At least by linking it to something pleasurable, you'll be creating incentive.

WATCH TALK SHOWS

This technique was contributed by one of my daughters, the same one who worries about what she's going to do when she has children if all they ever want to do is watch Oprah and eat junk food. She's convinced that a steady diet of the neurotic women on talk shows will make a person run to the gym for fear of turning into one of them. She reasons that a daily dose of fat women who hate skinny women, women who are willing to sell their first-born in order to afford liposuction, and women who make death threats on aerobic instructors should strike fear into the heart of anyone who has nothing better to do than watch these shows.

LIST THE PROS AND CONS OF WORKING OUT

This technique was contributed by another of my offspring. She suggests making two lists, one for the pros of working out and one for the cons. If the cons outweigh the pros, you don't have to go. Easy for her to say. She's under thirty, thinks water retention means putting the plug in the bathtub, and has the metabolism of a race horse.

Here's a sampling of her pros and cons:

Con: I'd rather stay home and watch TV.
Pro: If I work out, I'll have more energy to watch TV.
Con: Exercise is boring.
Pro: There are men at the gym.

Hopefully your lists will be more in depth and will convince you that over forty there aren't enough cons in the world to outweigh the pros of working out.

GET A DOG

Although not often regarded as a motivational tool, there is nothing like a dog to force you to exercise. Not a small, prissy dog that sits on the couch and picks fleas, but an active, pesky dog like a golden retriever or a lab that won't take no for an answer. If you refuse to take one of these dogs for a walk, it'll either jump on you, drag you off the couch with its teeth, or deposit lovely gifts on the carpet. (Not even a personal trainer will go to those lengths.) When it's bath time you'll do double-duty, and just try catching one of these animals when it's time to visit the vet. Spend enough hours with a dog or acquire more than one, and you'll probably be able to give up your health club membership.

HIRE A TRAINER

If you can afford to hire a private trainer, you won't have to worry about motivation. The trainer will do it for you. A skilled trainer will instruct you, monitor your progress, make sure you're doing things right, and more importantly, will push you through your workouts. The intensity of the one on one situation with someone watching your every move makes it virtually impossible for you to cheat or goof off.

Trainers come in a wide price range as well as in a variety of sizes, shapes, and personalities. Choose carefully. Observe them in action and ask around. Most can do the job for you, but there are a few types to watch out for:

The **baby sitter** treats you like a child, counting out your reps in a sing song voice and catering to your every need. Believe it or not, this can get old.

The **mother,** even more solicitous than the baby sitter, gives you tremendous guilt if you miss a workout and chicken soup if you're sick.

The **body buddy** (generally male) stands so close you feel as if he's doing your sets with you. He has his hands all over you which can be an unwelcome distraction, sexual harassment, or the biggest thrill of the day, depending on your point of view.

The **terrorist** has a booming voice and drill sergeant demeanor. He treats you like a dog and still believes in the "no pain, no gain" approach. He'll whip you into shape if he doesn't put you out of commission first.

The **socializer** knows and talks to everyone in the gym. You'll meet loads of new people but won't do five minutes worth of exercise.

COMPLAINING—AN UNDERRATED MOTIVATIONAL TECHNIQUE

Complaining is perhaps the most overlooked and underrated motivational technique. Proven to be dangerous and outdated, the old saying about "no pain, no gain," has been replaced by "gain without pain." It's my contention that it should be updated to "complain for gain." Complaining has been given a bad rap and has never really received the respect which it so richly deserves. Complaining can get you going and keep you moving when nothing else seems to work. Note that I'm referring to whole-hearted, honest-to-goodness bitching and not to mere whining, which is annoying and totally unacceptable.

Six Reasons that Complaining Is Good for Your Health

Reason #1. Complaining relieves stress.

Complaining is honest behavior which saves you from the stress of faking an attitude. You can express what you're really feeling instead of pretending that you're in a state of euphoria. Just think of the freedom when you can admit to yourself that you hate aerobics. You'll still have to take the classes, but you won't feel obligated to wear a mindless grin on your face.

Reason #2. Complaining releases negativity.

148

Complaining allows you to vent your negativity on the world instead of bottling it up and making yourself sick. Why hold back and get an ulcer, when revealing your true sentiments will allow you to feel so much better? If other people in the gym are getting on your nerves or if the place smells, get it off your chest. You may irritate everyone around you, but so what? They can simply turn around and complain about you.

Reason #3. Complaining saves you from martyrdom.

Suffering in silence is such a waste of time because it never engenders any sympathy. To the contrary, unless you're in the really big leagues, like Joan of Arc or my neighbor who baked for a charity event on the same day that she had her nails done, it's a major turnoff. Martyrs may go down in history, but they never get any respect in the gym.

Reason #4. Complaining increases your popularity.

Griping out loud can work wonders in enhancing your popularity because other women can relate to you. They understand where you're coming from, and they like you for it. You'd be amazed how quickly you can establish friendships and a true sense of camaraderie based on nothing more than mutual grievances.

Reason #5. Complaining makes you seem normal.

Exercising hard without grumbling arouses suspicion because it's abnormal. It causes people to shy away from you for fear that you're obsessive compulsive, anal retentive, or slightly deranged. You may not have much of a problem with this, but believe me it can get very lonely if the only time anyone ever talks to you is to share the name of a first rate shrink. By the way, save those names. You never can tell when they might come in handy.

Reason #6. Complaining distracts you.

Complaining is an easy way to keep your mind off what you're doing. If you find enough things to nit-pick about, you may forget your broader concerns about having to exercise in the first place. Let's say that against your better judgment, you've been coerced into going on a twenty-five mile bicycle ride. As you begin pedaling, you're worried about going the distance and about being stuck in the middle of nowhere trying to find a taxi, let alone a taxi with a bike rack. Then you realize how uncomfortable the seat is. Next it's the ugly helmet that gets your attention. Soon you're hot and thirsty and your bike shorts are riding up your crotch. Before you know it, you've gone the distance, and can spend the next two days bragging about the ride and moaning about how sore and tired you are.

Group Grouching—A New Approach

Group grouching is like a motivational party game. Quite simply, if several people are exercising together, they take turns announcing what's bothering them. It taps into creativity and competitiveness, while exposing you to complaints that you may never have thought of on your own.

Some friends of mine, who are definitely not well-conditioned athletes, used this technique while climbing 14,495 foot Mount Whitney, one of the highest mountains in the United States. Shocked to hear them planning this adventure, I asked them why they were making the trek (tactfully leaving out any mention of insanity). They gave me one of those "we're doing it because it's there" scenarios, but I didn't buy it for a second.

Awestruck when I heard that they'd completed their grueling mission, hiking from summer conditions at the bottom to virtual winter at the top, while wearing heavy backpacks (these are women who don't normally carry their own grocery bags), I had to know the secret of their success. At first they tried to throw me off the track by talking about training and discipline, but they finally admitted that it was complaining that had saved the day.

Whenever they felt as if they couldn't move another step, they'd try to one up each other on what was bothering them the most—no bathrooms, bugs, being stuck with each other on some godforsaken trail. When they were so unhappy that even this game lost its appeal, they took turns rating their relative distress (or their distressful relatives) on a scale of one to ten.

Popular Complaints You Can Use

If you're one of the miserable majority in the gym but are just too inhibited or too darn polite to express yourself—loosen up and try on a few of the following complaints for size:

- I should be getting paid to do this.
- I'm too (a) old (b) tired (c) intelligent for this.
- They ought to ban twenty year olds with boob jobs from the gym.
- My leotard is giving me a rash.
- My (fill in the body part) is killing me.
- I'm so hot, either the air conditioner is broken again or I've started the change.
- I have no energy. It must be my thyroid.
- This place smells like (a) a zoo (b) a barn (c) a men's room.
- I'm going to be sick. The pervert in the loose shorts is doing leg lifts again.
- I'd rather be (a) having a root canal (b) cleaning toilets (c) stuck in traffic.
- Exactly how expensive is liposuction?
- If I lift my thigh once more, my leg is going to fall off.
- And of course the old standby—there's got to be an easier way.

Chapter 15

Is that All There Is?

The Five
Extra Keys to Fitness

IS THAT ALL THERE IS?

Let's assume that desperation has driven you into a fitness lifestyle. You're doing the basics and have overcome the most common mistakes, but things aren't going the way you'd planned. You don't feel a day younger than you did when you started. Your corns still hurt, you're tired, and you continue to dread your workouts. You wonder why other women at the gym look as if they're at a party while you look as if you're on death row. You're getting so fed up that if things don't pick up soon, you're going to throw in the towel, go home and learn how to program your VCR. Wait! Don't do it! There's more.

There are five elements which, when added to the fitness basics, will turn you from an exercise drone to an exercise diva; from an aging mess to an aging miracle. If you're thinking luck, favorable genetics, and plastic surgery you wouldn't be wrong. However, I'm referring to five intangibles which are safe, painless, and readily available at no extra charge. All you have to do is tap into your own energy and resourcefulness to find these life enhancing qualities.

I like to think of them as the psychological keys to fitness, the factors that will make the difference between going through the motions and really getting results. It's as if two people were learning to dance and one meticulously followed a series of footprints on the floor, while the other put on a cute outfit, listened to the music and let her body move to the beat. They'd both learn how to do it, but the second dancer would get more joy out of the process and be a much bigger hit at parties.

THE FIVE EXTRA KEYS TO FITNESS

1. ATTITUDE

Attitude, the first key, encompasses the way you think, act, and feel about yourself and about life in general. It's reflected in everything you do from the way you carry yourself to the way you wear your hair. Attitude is not something you can easily hide, although people have been known to fake it.

Slouching into a gym as if you're trying to disappear won't prevent people from noticing you. To the contrary, they'll ask themselves, "Who was that insecure person who just slouched by?" No matter what your

154

age or physical condition, you have to develop an attitude that says "I'm tough and can do whatever I set my mind to." You have to stand up and be counted, not hang back and be intimidated.

If you're overweight but attempting to remedy the problem, be proud when you walk into a health club. At least you're making an effort rather than sitting at home wallowing in self-pity and ice cream. If you stay on a bike for fifteen minutes, even though you feel as if you're on the last leg of the Tour de France, pat yourself on the back instead of putting yourself down for not doing more.

This positive mind set is an integral part of each successful exercise session. Getting into the right attitude is almost more important than getting into the right leotard and tights. If you drag your way through a workout, it'll be a chore and you'll hate every second of it. But if you can manage to throw yourself into it with some energy (even if you complain every step of the way), the time will go faster and you'll feel much more satisfied when it's over.

An attitude problem for many older women is the belief that they're past their prime so they may as well give up. They step over the forty threshold and close themselves off to new experiences. They trade in a sense of adventure for support hose and a pair of orthopedic shoes. "I'm too old for this" becomes their rallying cry. Who says you're too old for anything? Is there a committee that marks arbitrary cutoff points for what you can and cannot do? Granted, there are physical limitations, but a negative attitude shouldn't be the deciding factor. If you choose to be old and unfit, you'll be old and unfit. If you elect to savor life and experience it to the fullest, you'll be young and vibrant no matter what your birth certificate or anyone else says.

Closely related to the "I'm too old for this" group are the "settlers." These are women who have achieved their goals—husband, children, careers, etc.—basically accomplished what they set out to do and are now content to rest on their laurels. The irony is that most of them aren't content and often echo the words of that depressing Peggy Lee song, "Is that all there is?" They're bored and dissatisfied because they're living with the safety of what they know and have already experienced instead of opening themselves up to new adventures. They've put artificial limitations on themselves based on nothing more than age and low expectations. You don't have to jump out of a plane to put some zest back into your existence (unless you're completely out of your mind), but at least continue to challenge yourself. Don't let your life go on without you.

Another issue which can often be resolved with a change in attitude is a lack of self-esteem. Far too many older women downgrade their accomplishments, failing to recognize their self-worth. They fall victim to a society which judges success in monetary terms and overlooks the value of personal achievements. This negativity carries over into other aspects of their lives, including eating and exercise habits.

Life Résumé

I used to be a prime example. Whenever anyone would ask "What do you do?" I'd be at a loss because I wasn't sure if any of my activities were significant enough to mention. Then one evening during my domestic phase, when my husband wanted to know why I was taking a class on making radish roses, I defensively blurted out, "I'm adding to my life résumé." I had no idea what I was talking about, but neither did my husband, so it worked.

Upon reflection, I realized the validity of what I'd said. Writing a life résumé is a way to acknowledge the value of your various pursuits. If you give yourself credit for everything you've ever done—each job, class, volunteer position, and personal achievement—you'll be amazed at your versatility.

Consider internal accomplishments as well as external—the ways that you've developed and grown throughout your lifetime. Do you embrace challenges instead of running from them as you might have in the past? Have you made positive changes in yourself or at least learned to enjoy your faults? Have you found an inner peace that previously eluded you? These feats are every bit as valuable as anything else you may have done.

Give yourself enough credit and you'll wonder how a person of your abilities could ever have been so unsure of herself. You'll see that increasing self-esteem doesn't necessarily require major life changes. It may simply be a matter of revising your attitude toward what you've already achieved.

2. PASSION

Passion, the next key to fitness, is often what gets you into bed, but it may also be just what it takes to get you out of bed in the morning. Find a passion for something in your life. Note that was **something** not someone. Of course it's thrilling to feel passion for another human being, but that passion is dependent on someone else's feelings. If unrequited, it may be more aggravation than it's worth. On the other hand, if it's mutual, it can restore youthfulness and vitality.

Ideally, we would all have a passion for life itself, but it doesn't always work that way. There are too many days when you ask yourself, "What's the point? Why shave under my arms and put on deodorant for this?" The point is that you have to find something that gets your juices flowing, that rekindles your excitement for being alive, that fills you with a sense of anticipation.

Have you ever seen people bird watching or fishing and asked yourself, "How can they spend so much time doing something so boring?" The answer is that they love what they're doing, or, as in the case of fishing, may have fallen asleep. They become so engrossed in the activity that they lose track of time and place.

Some lucky people have a true passion for their work. It's absorbing, fulfilling, and makes them come alive. While others, who think they have a passion for their work because it's so all-consuming, are really type A personalities who can't function on any other level. They're mistaking compulsion for passion. If you fall into the first category, consider yourself blessed. If you fall into the second, get a relaxing hobby before job stress kills you.

Feel free to groan at what I'm about to write because it's very corny, but it's also true. Women with passion have a sparkle in their eyes and more energy in their step. They have a love affair with life that translates into a healthy self-love.

3. HUMOR

Humor is not often mentioned in regard to fitness, but for me it's as much a part of being healthy as breathing in and out. It's one of the most effective means of defusing tension, counteracting frustration, and coping with life's little one-two punches. Humor can lead to rejuvenated physical and mental well-being by letting you experience the same carefree laughter that you did when you were a child.

There's nothing like a deep down, shake all over belly laugh to relieve stress. It allows you to put your problems on hold, to take time out from being uptight and overly controlled, and to let your hair down without worrying about how silly you look.

After a great laugh, you often feel pleasantly exhausted, relaxed, content, and ready to move on, the same as you do after a great workout or great sex. Laughter, however, is less complicated than sex because you're assured that everyone involved is having as much fun as you are. You can be equally gratified with or without a partner, and you can do it in public without getting arrested.

Have you ever noticed how some people laugh when they're nervous, generally at inopportune moments when their giggling is blatantly obvious to everyone within earshot? Despite the fact that people who don't understand this sort of inadvertent behavior find it incredibly offensive, it works wonders in dispelling tension. I know, because I've laughed at overly formal dinner parties where I was supposed to make a favorable impression (I didn't), and if the truth be known, at a funeral or two.

Humor is also an effective tool for counteracting frustration. The ability to take yourself less seriously gives you the freedom to make mistakes and to forgive yourself if you're not perfect (although I am, so that's not an issue for me). Remember, a primary reason for working out is to feel better about yourself, so lighten up and enjoy it.

Certainly there are times when you're bound to give in to depression or anxiety, but there are also times that would seem less dismal if you could view them from a more humorous perspective. Laughter may not eliminate a problem, but it can make you better able to cope with it.

For instance, when you're struggling through an aerobics class and some young thing is giving you a hard time about "invading her space," don't get upset. Instead, helpfully mention that her tights are wrinkled in the back and suggest that she might want to straighten them out. In the next breath, correct yourself with great chagrin and mutter, "Oops, I didn't realize you weren't wearing any." She may not laugh, but you will. When you're out to dinner and the snotty young waiter inquires if you'd like him to turn on the overhead lights and bring you a magnifying glass so that you can read the menu, don't get insulted. Instead, tell yourself how amusing it's going to be when you don't leave him a tip.

The aging process is inevitable. There's nothing inherently funny about it, but accepting it with humor helps to take the edge off. In the words of the poet W.H. Auden, "Laughter is both an act of protest and an act of acceptance." This applies so well to growing older because most of us stage all sorts of protests, but in the end we have no recourse but to laugh at the sick jokes of Father Time. And make no mistake about that, it is Father Time. This system is definitely not the brainchild of a female mind. Now senility is another matter. It would take a woman's brilliant touch to realize that when you can no longer fight the ravages of aging, it's in your own best interest to be oblivious to them.

For those of you who are worried about laugh lines, which some misguided fools say give the face character, but which certainly don't make it look any younger, here's a tip from my in-house experts. When you feel a laugh coming on, purse your lips and hoot like an owl. In theory, this prevents you from scrunching up your face and adding nasty wrinkles.

Give it a try, although I must tell you, it never worked for me. Aside from being unsatisfying, it looked and sounded so ridiculous that it made me laugh until I had tears rolling down my face and wrinkles lined up just waiting to happen.

4. INSTINCT

According to the dictionary, instinct is "a natural feeling, knowledge, or power, such as that which guides animals; an inborn tendency to act in a certain way." As the fourth key to fitness, instinct is the ability to listen to these inborn feelings and innate knowledge, to hear what your body is screaming at you. This doesn't require ESP, an interpreter, or even a personal trainer. It's simply a matter of paying attention to your gut reactions so that you stop fighting your natural rhythms and inclinations.

In the words of Charles Darwin, "The very essence of an instinct is that it is followed independently of reason." Because the human mind is more complex than those of other animals, we frequently spend so much time analyzing, that we overlook our basic responses. When a bird builds a nest, it doesn't agonize over blueprints and neighborhood. It merely heeds a natural call and gets the job done. For many women, the concept of listening to their own bodies is so foreign that if they were birds, they'd end up laying their eggs on the sidewalk.

It's easy to get so caught up in following a prescribed fitness regimen, in "doing the right thing," that you don't pay attention to how it's really affecting you. Locked into your goals, you make the common mistake of overtraining, with only a vague sense that you're doing anything wrong. You ignore the warning signs until it's too late, and you end up on the missing- in-exercise-action list. I don't care how individualized your program may be, it won't work unless you're in tune with your body.

Obviously, if you have to be removed from the gym on a stretcher, you're overdoing it, but you can be alerted to excess in more subtle ways. Too many nagging aches or pains, chronic exhaustion, insomnia, flagging enthusiasm, weight problems, nightmares about fluorescent jogging suits, chills at the sight of a fitness infomercial—these are all signs that your body is trying to get in touch with you.

Listening to your instincts allows you to differentiate between true burnout and plain old laziness. On any given day, if you experience excessive difficulty in getting into a routine, give yourself about fifteen minutes. If things really don't improve (be honest), stop exercising and go home. This doesn't mean that you should pack it in if you don't burst into the gym like Richard Simmons on speed (what a horrifying thought). But once you get warmed up and your endorphins kick in, your level of energy should increase, and you should almost start to enjoy what you're doing. I suppose that puts you in danger of becoming an endorphin junkie, but it sure beats becoming a lazy, guilt-ridden, out of shape exercise dropout.

Biorhythms

Being aware of your natural biorhythms, which are simply cycles of change in the functioning of an organism, is another way in which your instincts can pay off. There are researchers who go so far as to suggest that we regularly go through three cycles—physical, emotional, and intellectual—which can be used to predict day to day variations in feelings and in the ability to perform physical and mental tasks. Some scientists claim that these biorhythms occur independently. Others believe that they're related to external cycles, such as the tides and the phases of the moon.

No matter what causes these normal fluctuations, recognizing them will allow you to exercise more efficiently. If you're in a low cycle, feeling out of synch and unable to get anything accomplished, give yourself a break and keep your training goals modest. If you're in an up cycle, expect a little more from yourself—walk a bit further or lift a few extra pounds (that's lift, not gain).

If you have any doubt about the whole theory of biorhythms, consider that it offers a perfect rationalization for mood swings, bloating, mental lapses, and essentially anything else that you haven't got an excuse for. Keeping a fitness journal, as I discussed earlier, will further convince you because over the course of time you'll see a gradually emerging picture of your own built-in cycles.

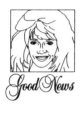

The longer and more consistently you work out and stick with a fitness lifestyle, the better you'll come to know your body. You'll learn to listen to and trust your instincts. Taking care of yourself will become a sure thing instead of a crap shoot. You'll know when to sleep, how much to eat, and how hard to push yourself. Once you've got the basics down, it'll be easy to assimilate or discard the hottest new fitness tip of the week. Instead of becoming a walking target for fad diets and trendy exercise regimens, you'll be confident of your own needs. You may even be able to get that nest off the sidewalk and back into a tree.

5. ILLUSION

I have my paternal grandmother (not the shrinking one) to thank for opening my eyes to illusion, the last but far from least of the five keys. She used to say, "Stand up straight, walk fast, and no one will be able to tell how old you really are." I can remember her at eighty-something, strutting around at breakneck pace in size four, high-heeled shoes. She may have had gray hair and a fair share of wrinkles but she was right, from her posture and speed, you'd never have guessed her age. Besides, you could barely get a glance at her face as she whizzed by.

Illusion is the art of accentuating your assets and concealing your flaws so that you look even better than you really do. (Does that make any sense whatsoever?) Working out to improve your health may be vital, but it's certainly not as motivational as working out to improve your appearance. I guarantee you most women would spend fewer hours exercising if no one was ever going to view the results. It's for the same reason that the famous Gold's Gym originated in sunny southern California instead of Alaska.

Looking your best gives you an added measure of confidence, a psychological edge, that allows you to do your finest work. Think about it. On those days when you don't wash your hair, forgo makeup, and throw on whatever drops out of the closet, you probably couldn't even talk your way out of a traffic ticket (not that I'm speaking from personal experience).

Let me phrase it another way. Would you like to spend the entire day looking like you do when you first fall out of bed in the morning, or are you thankful that you can give yourself a boost? As for me, if that first glance in the mirror was as good as it was going to get, I'd put a paper bag over my head.

Tools of Illusion

The following are a few basic tools for creating illusion.

Makeup. When you're young and gorgeous without dark circles, lines, and age spots, you probably don't require much more enhancement than a dab of moisturizer. But when you reach the age when soaking your head in a vat of moisturizer wouldn't be overkill, it's time for a cosmetic pick-me-up. If you're not sure what shades go best with aging skin, stop in at your local department store. Most cosmetic counters offer a free makeup session in an effort to ring up sales.

Ignore so called friends who tell you how much prettier you are "au naturale." They're trying to throw you off the track because they're jealous. As for men who claim to prefer unadorned faces, they're jealous too because they don't have all of our options for self-enhancement. They may also be trying to score a few extra points.

When it comes to hair coloring, it's certainly your prerogative to show off the grays if you're so inclined, but my question is—why? You might as well place a little sign on your forehead reading, "Guess what. I'm older than I look." If you're the rare woman who loves her gray hair, be careful with those blue and purple tints. Unless you're able to pull off a punk look (which is doubtful), people will assume you're too far gone to care.

Clothing. Clothing, like makeup, is an invaluable tool in creating illusion. A modicum of common sense will enable you to select garments that emphasize the positive and camouflage the rest. If you have a great pair of legs but your arms are a work in progress, shorten your skirts and forget sleeveless blouses. To the contrary, if you've toned your upper body by working out, but your legs haven't received the message, bare more of the top and wear well-tailored slacks or longer skirts. If your once treasured chest has turned to sunken treasure, rethink the strapless items in your wardrobe.

Consider that vertical stripes create a longer, leaner impression, while horizontal stripes add width, particularly around the hips. If you're excessively overweight, experiment with softly shaped garments instead of baggy numbers, which may actually make you seem heavier. Gathers and shoulder pads can also add pounds.

If you're not sure if an outfit works for you, stand in front of a mirror and pretend you're looking at a stranger. See what comments leap to mind.

One of the greatest advances in the field of illusory clothing is what I refer to as "orthopedic underwear." These magical garments, like the Wonder Bra, take what you've got and temporarily put it back where it used to be. They can slim your waist, shape your butt, and even bring you the miracle of cleavage.

If this type of underwear makes you look so fabulous that you can't see the need for exercise, bear in mind what happens when you take it off. Your bra and panties may not be the only things to hit the floor.

Warning

Posture. Standing up straight and sucking in your gut can do more for your appearance than a year on the treadmill. Half the trick with diet and exercise ads that feature "before" and "after" photos (aside from no makeup and bad hair) is carriage. In the "before," the women are often slouched over with bellies sagging, while in the "after" they're standing as if a broomstick has been placed in an unfortunate location. No wonder they look like two different people. Try it in front of a mirror and see the illusion for yourself.

According to the American Physical Therapy Association, there are three elements to proper posture:

- A healthy back with its three natural curves
- Strong musculature
- Flexible joints

Far be it from me to overstate the obvious, but stretching and weight lifting are two of the best ways to achieve those results. The third is to become aware of the way you're carrying yourself.

Freeze in place right now and note how you're standing or sitting. If you're drooping, repeat five times, "this makes me look older and less attractive." Then, straighten up. If your abdomen is protruding, suck it in and hold it tight. Do this test several times a day, and you'll quickly discover how often you let it all hang out and how easy it is to remedy the situation. As a bonus, you'll be strengthening muscles with a minimum of effort.

Hint

Weights. Weight training allows you to create an illusion by reshaping your proportions—using lighter weights to tone and tighten selected areas and heavier weights to build others. For example, if you're big-boned with large hips, you may not be able to make those hips disappear (which seems highly unfair when you consider that certain magicians can make airplanes disappear), but you can make them seem smaller by increasing the size of your shoulders. By the same token, if you're an alien life form whose hips and legs are too small, you can work to increase their size while maintaining the tone of your upper body.

PUTTING IT ALL TOGETHER

The tricks of illusion when combined with the right attitude, passion, a sense of humor, and the ability to follow your instincts will put you so far ahead of the game that you may be tempted to skip exercising and eating right altogether. Don't even think about it! The fitness basics—aerobic exercise, weight training, stretching, and proper nutrition—are essential for turning the old you into the newer model. Put it all together, the basics plus the extras, and you'll look better, feel better, and be able to lie about your age forever.

Chapter 16

In Conclusion

Aging, to borrow an expression from my trio of daughters, "sucks." It's also inevitable. The trick to coping with the ups and downs of the aging process is to consider the alternative and realize that getting older is your best option. Focus on the positives such as acquired wisdom (which I'm assuming will kick in any day now), being comfortable with yourself, and coming into your own. Hopefully, this positive thinking will override your concerns about fading skin, falling body parts, and hair that grows where it shouldn't and falls out where it's supposed to grow.

Once you've accepted the fact that you're going to age, you can take some decisive action and do it with flair. Follow the advice I've offered in this book, and you'll age like fine wine instead of going flat in the can like stale beer. A simple fitness lifestyle, the basics enhanced by the five extras, is the way to retain what you've got for as long as possible. It requires some effort, but it's much more empowering than sitting back and letting nature take its course.

It's not always easy to pass up chocolate cake for a carrot stick or to pass up a white sale for an aerobics class, but self-discipline does have its rewards. You'll look better, you'll feel better, you won't seem as ridiculous when you dress inappropriately for your age, and you'll receive tons of compliments. As an added incentive, the older you get the more incredible people will think you are for staying in shape. Hit the gym when you're eighty, and you'll get the kind of respect that's generally reserved for women like Eleanor Roosevelt (who, by the way, would probably have benefited from a little exercise program).

Women who incorporate the fitness basics into their lifestyles are stronger and more vital. They have more energy during the day and enjoy more restful sleep at night. To top it all off, they have better sex lives which, of course, means that they get better jewelry.

Staying fit requires some sacrifice, but remember, you can complain all you like while you're doing it. Not being gung ho or developing a positive mental attitude about exercising and eating right doesn't mean that you're a failure. As I assured you in the beginning of the book, it simply means that you're normal.

Besides, you have something special working in your favor, something that no one under the age of forty can truly appreciate. You're desperate.

Being desperate will keep you going when all else fails. So take that big step. Come out of the closet, proudly admit that you're desperate, and join the millions of other women who feel exactly the same way you do. There's strength in numbers, and when those numbers are made up of women on the edge, there's no limit to what can be accomplished.

No more lame excuses. No more hiding under baggy clothes. Put down this book. Throw out the ice cream you have hidden in the back of the freezer. Call a desperate friend and make a date to go walking first thing tomorrow morning.

GLOSSARY

Aerobic exercise—Continuous exercise of the large muscle groups that raises your heart rate, causes you to sweat like a pig (not to be confused with glow), makes you tired and sore, and is nowhere near as much fun as sex

Basal metabolic rate—Level of energy required to perform vital functions such as respiration and repair

Cardiovascular fitness—Healthy heart and blood vessels

Ectomorph—Someone with a long and lean physique

Endomorph—Someone with a more fatty physique

Endorphins—Natural pain suppressants released by the brain when certain nerves are stimulated; like taking drugs, only safer and more cost effective

Fitness organizations
    ACE—American Council on Exercise
    ACSM—American College of Sports Medicine
    AFAA—Aerobics and Fitness Association of America

High impact—More forceful activities that may involve jumping or pounding movements and thus put increased strain on the body

Low impact—Usually non-jarring activities that are easier on the joints and on the bladder

Mesomorph—Someone with a naturally muscular physique

Osteoporosis—A progressive disease that causes bone tissue to deteriorate until the bones are so weak and brittle that they break under the slightest strain

Repetition—Cycle of lifting a weight and returning it to the starting point

Set—A group of repetitions

Spot reducing—A myth

Training zone—Exercise pace that will burn fat and improve the cardiovascular system without overtaxing it